HEALING YOUR THYROID NATURALLY WITH AYURVEDA

HEALING THE THYROID NATURALLY

Dr. Ajay Kumar
BAMS, M.D.(KC),BHU, Ph.D.(KC),BHU
Asst.Professor, Deptt. Of Kayachikitsa
Govt. PG Ayurveda College & Hospital
Varanasi

Dr. Pratima Yadav
BAMS, M.D.(Panchakarma)
Govt. PG Ayurveda College & Hospital, Varanasi
Medical Officer, U.P. Government

ATREYA HEALTH SERIES

NOTION PRESS

India. Singapore. Malaysia.

HEALING THE THYROID NATURALLY

Published by Notion Press 2025

ISBN:

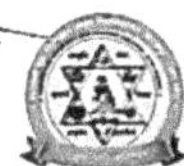
MAHAYOGI GURU GORAKHNATH AYUSH UNIVERSITY
Bhatahat, Gorakhpur Uttar Pradesh, India

Prof. Dr. A.K. Singh
Vice-Chancellor
Mob.: 96300-31233
vc.ayushuniversitygkp@gmail.com

Temp. Office: I.A.S./P.C.S. Coaching Centre
Near Prem Chand Park, Narmal Campus, Gorakhpur-273001
vc@mggaugkp.ac.in www.mggaugkp.ac.in
Office No.: 0551-2989819

Date: 18.01.2025

FOREWORD

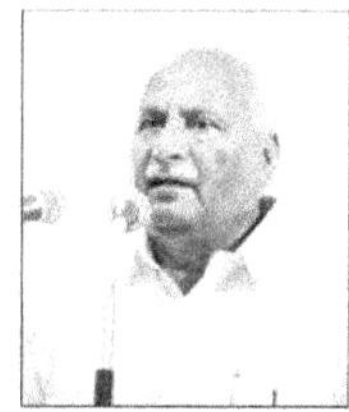

The thyroid gland, a small yet powerful organ located in the neck, plays a crucial role in maintaining the body's metabolism, energy levels, and overall well-being. Despite its significance, thyroid disorders have become alarmingly common in modern times, often linked to stress, environmental toxins, poor dietary habits, and lifestyle imbalances. For many, the diagnosis of a thyroid condition can feel overwhelming, leading to a lifetime of dependence on medications or invasive procedures. However, there exists an ancient, time-tested path that can offer hope, healing, and sustainable solutions - Ayurveda.

'Healing the Thyroid Naturally' is a transformative guide that bridges the timeless principles of Ayurveda with the needs of the modern individual. This book goes beyond conventional approaches to thyroid health, inviting readers to explore the root causes of their imbalances and empowering them to embrace natural, holistic methods for restoration. It is a reminder that true healing is not just about addressing symptoms but about nurturing the body, mind, and spirit as an integrated whole. The ancient science of Ayurveda teaches us that every individual is unique, governed by their distinct constitution, or prakriti, which is determined by the interplay of the three doshas - vata, pitta, and kapha. This personalized approach to health lies at the heart of Ayurveda's effectiveness in managing thyroid disorders.

Through this book, readers will discover how imbalances in these doshas manifest in the thyroid and learn how to harmonize their body's natural rhythms through diet, herbal remedies, detoxification, yoga, meditation, and lifestyle changes. The all authors have skilfully distilled complex Ayurvedic concepts into practical insights, making this book accessible to both beginners and seasoned practitioners. Drawing on years of research, clinical experience, and a deep understanding of holistic healing, the authors provide actionable steps to address conditions such as hypothyroidism, hyperthyroidism, and other related imbalances. Each chapter is thoughtfully designed to guide readers through their healing journey, from understanding the thyroid's role in the body to implementing Ayurvedic practices tailored to their individual needs.

One of the most valuable aspects of this book is its emphasis on prevention and long-term well-being. The authors not only address the management of existing thyroid conditions but also highlights ways to strengthen and support thyroid health for a lifetime. Readers will find detailed descriptions of medicinal herbs, step-by-step detoxification protocols, and practical tips for cultivating mental and emotional resilience.

Healing the Thyroid Naturally is more than a book - it is a call to action for those seeking to reclaim their health and vitality. It is a testament to the wisdom of Ayurveda and its profound ability to heal and transform lives. For anyone who has felt the frustration of conventional treatments or yearned for a deeper connection to their own body, this book offers a beacon of hope and a roadmap to holistic wellness.

As you embark on this journey through the pages of this remarkable work, I encourage you to embrace the principles shared here with an open heart and mind. Trust in the ancient wisdom of Ayurveda, and let it guide you toward balance, harmony, and healing. May this book inspire you to take charge of your health, rediscover your inner strength, and live a life of vibrant well-being.

With best wishes,

(Prof. A.K. Singh)
Vice-Chancellor
Mahayogi Guru Gorakhnath AYUSH University,
Gorakhpur,
Uttar Pradesh

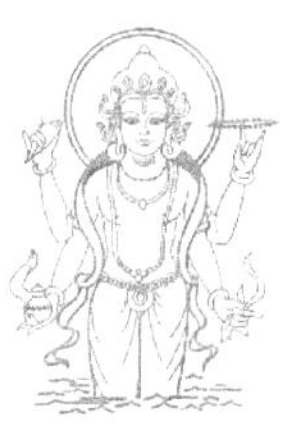

PREFACE

For centuries, Ayurveda, the ancient Indian system of medicine, has offered profound insights into the intricate workings of the human body and mind. This time-honoured tradition recognizes that true health extends far beyond the mere absence of disease, encompassing a harmonious balance of physical, mental, and emotional well-being. At the heart of this holistic approach lies the understanding that each individual is unique, possessing a distinct constitution – a combination of doshas (bio-energies) that govern their physical, mental, and emotional characteristics. This inherent individuality necessitates a personalized approach to healthcare, where treatment plans are tailored to address the specific needs and imbalances of each person.

This book, "***Healing the Thyroid Naturally***," delves into the profound wisdom of this ancient system to explore the intricate relationship between the thyroid gland and the delicate equilibrium of the doshas. The thyroid, a small but mighty gland situated at the base of the neck, plays a crucial role in regulating various bodily functions, including metabolism, energy levels, mood, and overall well-being.

When this vital organ falls out of balance, it can manifest as a range of debilitating symptoms, from fatigue and weight fluctuations to anxiety and hormonal disruptions.

Conventional medicine often relies on a one-size-fits-all approach to managing thyroid conditions, primarily through medication. However, many individuals seek natural and holistic alternatives to address the root causes of their imbalances and reclaim their vitality. Ayurveda offers a compassionate and personalized pathway to healing, focusing on nourishing the body, calming the mind, and cultivating inner balance.

Within these pages, you will embark on a journey of self-discovery, learning to:

- Understand the Ayurvedic perspective on the thyroid: Explore how Ayurveda views the thyroid gland within the context of the interconnectedness of the body's systems.
- Identify your unique constitution (Dosha): Delve into the intricacies of your individual dosha composition and understand how it influences your susceptibility to thyroid imbalances.
- Nourish your thyroid with Ayurvedic principles: Discover a wide array of natural remedies, including dietary guidelines, herbal formulations, and lifestyle modifications specifically tailored to support thyroid health and restore balance to the doshas.
- Embody mind-body practices for optimal thyroid function: Explore

the transformative power of yoga, meditation, and pranayama (breathwork) in calming the mind, reducing stress, and optimizing thyroid function.

- Create a personalized healing plan: Learn to integrate Ayurvedic principles into your daily life to support long-term thyroid health and cultivate a vibrant sense of well-being.

This book is not intended to be a substitute for professional medical advice. It is designed to empower you with valuable knowledge and tools to work collaboratively with your healthcare provider to optimize your thyroid health and embark on a journey of holistic healing.

May this book serve as a guide on your path to reclaiming your vitality and experiencing the profound benefits of Ayurveda in supporting your thyroid and overall well-being.

Date: 02.02.2025 Warmly,

(Basant Panchami)

AKumar

(Dr Ajay Kumar)

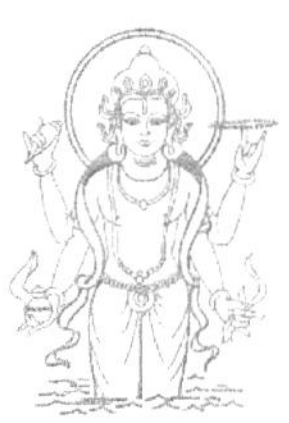

ACKNOWLEDGMENTS

This book is a culmination of years of study, research, and clinical experience. It would not have been possible without the support and guidance of many individuals.

First and foremost, I express my deepest gratitude to my teachers and mentors, whose wisdom and compassion have profoundly shaped my understanding of Ayurveda. Their dedication to the healing arts has been an inspiration.

I am immensely grateful to my family and friends for their unwavering support, encouragement, and understanding throughout this journey. Their love and belief in me have been a constant source of strength.

I would also like to thank the countless patients who have entrusted me with their health and shared their stories. Their courage, resilience, and unwavering hope have been a constant source of inspiration.

A special thanks to Junior Residents of Department of Kayachikitsa & Panchakarma. Their Exclusive Support and dedication have been invaluable in bringing this book to execution.

Finally, I extend my heartfelt gratitude to all those who have contributed to the rich and vibrant tradition of Ayurveda. This book is a testament to the enduring wisdom and healing power of this ancient system of medicine.

Warmly,

(Dr Ajay Kumar)

आदिदेव भगवान धन्वंतरि

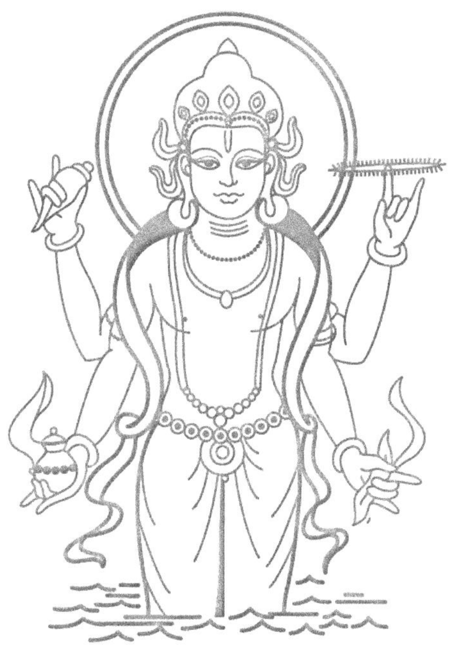

नमामि धन्वंतरिमादि देवं सुराः सुरैर्वन्दित पाद पद्मम् ।
लोकैर्जरारुक् भय मृत्यु नाशं धातारमिशंविविधौषधिनाम् ॥१॥
चंव्योमवातावनिवारिवहिं पंच प्रपंचात्मक देहभाजम् ।
संताप संपात जरा ज्वरान्तकं नमामि धन्वंतरिमादि देवम् ॥२॥
नवीन नील मुदकान्ति कान्तं शान्तं हरैर्द्वादशमाख्यमूर्तिम् ।
पूर्ति शतानां सुमनोरथानां नमामि धन्वंतरिमादि देवम् ॥३॥

INDEX

1.Thyroid: Ayurvedic Perspective **1**

Historical Review 7

Involvement Of Agni in Hypothyroidism 8

Status Of Ama in Hypothyroidism 10

Clinical Conditions Similar to Hypothyroidism 14

Types Of Galgand 23

Chikitsa (Treatment) 25

2.Thyroid Anatomy **27**

Blood Supply 31

Venous Drainage 32

Nerve Supply 32

Function Of Thyroid Gland 32

3.Hypothyroidism: A Brief Overview **35**

Etiology Of Hypothyroidism 36

Clinical Manifestations 37

Diagnosis Of Hypothyroidism 39

Management Of Hypothyroidism 41

Complications Of Hypothyroidism 42

Myxedema Coma 42

Subclinical Hypothyroidism 43

4.Hyperthyroidism: Brief Review **51**

Symptoms Of Hyperthyroidism 52

Diagnosis Of Hyperthyroidism 54

Diet And Hyperthyroidism: A Deeper Dive 58
Treatment For Hyperthyroidism 60
Ayurvedic Treatment for Hyperthyroidism 63
5.Gestational Hypothyroidism 69
Effect Of Pregnancy on Thyroid Physiology 71
Physiological Changes During Pregnancy 74
Iodine Requirement in Pregnancy 75
Classification Of Gestational Hypothyroidism 77
Symptoms Of Gestational Hypothyroidism 78
Management Of Gestational Hypothyroidism 84
6.Balancing Your Thyroid 93
Subclinical Hypothyroidism (Sch) 94
The Ayurvedic Perspective 94
Ayurvedic Treatment Strategies 95
Comprehensive Ayurvedic Treatment 96
Detoxification Through Panchakarma 96
Lifestyle Adjustments for Thyroid Health 97
A Closer Look at Herbal Remedies 99
Ayurvedic Formulations 103
7.Panchakarma in Thyroid Disorder 105
Vamana (Emesis Therapy) 105
Virechana (Purgation Therapy) 106
Basti (Enema Therapy) 106
Nasya (Nasal Administration) 106

Raktamokshana (Blood Letting Therapy) 107
Benefits Of Panchakarma 108
Nasya Karma 110
8.Drugs For Thyroid Disorders 135
Kanchanar 137
Shunthi 140
Nimba 143
Ashwagandha 146
Bacopa 148
Nigella Sativa 151
Turmeric 154
Guggul 157
Punarnava 160
9.Nutrients For Healthy Thyroid 163
Iodine 163
Selenium 165
Zinc 166
Vitamin D 168
Vitamin B12 169
Magnesium 170
Tyrosine 171
Iron 172
10.Foods For Healthy Thyroid 175
Why Diet Matters For Thyroid Health 175

Foods That Should Be Avoided 176
Foods That Can Be Eaten 177
11.Yoga For Hypothyroidism 181
Ujjayi Pranayama 182
Halasana 184
Sarvangasana 186
Bhujangasana 187
12.Research & Case Studies 191
Ayurvedic Treatment Principles 192
Case Study – 1 193
Case Study - 2 196
Case Study - 3 199
Case Study - 4 208
Case Study - 5 213
Conclusions From the Case Studies 218

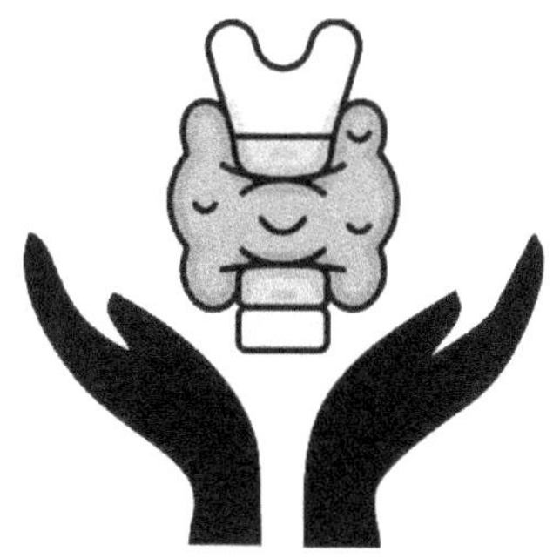

Thyroid: Ayurvedic Perspective

Dr. Ajay Kumar, Dr. Pratima Yadav

Ayurveda is an ancient Indian system of medicine, which stresses principally on prevention of body ailments rather than simply relieving pathological problems or symptoms. The sign and symptoms of hypothyroidism are similar to those of *Kapha Vriddhi, Rasa Dushti, Meda Dushti, Meda Dhatvagni Mandya*. The treatment modalities of hypothyroidism are also having many adverse effects, so it is the need of time to look for a safe and effective treatment for hypothyroidism in **Ayurveda**. To make an effective treatment, the disease hypothyroidism should be understood in terms of **Ayurveda** principle.

Hypothyroidism results in slowing of metabolic process and energy expenditure. It results in a many of clinical signs and symptoms. The *Kapha* symptoms like lethargy, sleepiness, weight gain, decreased appetite, cold intolerance, fullness in the throat, hoarseness of voice, etc. are produced. The *Vata* symptoms like fatigue, loss of energy, dry skin, hair loss, muscle pain, joint pain, weakness in the extremities, mental impairment, forgetfulness, impaired memory, inability to concentrate, blurred vision, decreased hearing, constipation, menstrual disturbances, impaired fertility, decreased perspiration. These all symptoms are produced due to increment of *Kapha-Vata* mainly. Vitiation of *Doshas* also depends on vitiations of *Agni* and therefore **Acharya Vagbhat** has said that

रोगाः सर्वेऽपि मन्देऽग्नौ सुतरामुदराणि तु।। अ.हृ.नि. 12/1

which means, Pathophysiology of all diseases lies in the concept of *Agni*, as *Agni* is said to be the *Prana* (life) of the living body. Also, body is made up of *Dosha, Dhatu*, & *Mala.*

दोषधातुमलमूलं हि शरीरं।

Nourishment of each of these solely depends on balanced *Agni* of each *Dhatu.* As said by **Acharya Charak**

आयुर्वर्णबलं स्वास्थ्यमुत्साहोपचयौ प्रभा।
ओजस्तेजोऽग्न्यः प्राणाश्चोक्ता देहाग्निहेतुकाः।। च.चि. 15/33

Vitiation of *Srotas* also depends on *Agni.* So, it is clear that in hypothyroidism there is abnormality of *Agni* with abnormality of *Kapha* and *Vata Doshas* as well as *Rasavaha, Raktavaha, Medovaha, Shukravaha* and *Manovaha Srotas.*

The main treatment of hypothyroidism in modern medicine is hormone replacement therapy (HRT). But hormone (levothyroxine) has to be taken lifelong and has certain side effects on long term use. It can cause cardiac arrhythmias, precipitate angina, palpitation, osteoporosis etc. The adverse effects of HRT and increasing prevalence of hypothyroidism compels for the need of safer modalities of treatment which are equally effective and have lesser side effects. According to sign and symptoms the hypothyroidism is purely Kapha-Vata Vyadhi.

Hypothyroidism is one of the earliest endocrine gland disorders after diabetes. Hypothyroidism is the second most prevailing disorders in day-to-day practice. The reason of hypothyroidism may be due to our lifestyle change like dietary, sedentary habits and lack of exercise. In the current highly civilized era, stress of day-to-day life along with irregular food habits and sedentary life style affect one's bodily organs through several psycho-somatic mechanisms. This has resulted in various metabolic disorders. Among these disorders, hypothyroidism is significant for its increasing incidence.

Hypothyroidism is a clinical syndrome resulting from deficiency of thyroid hormones due to their insufficient synthesis which in turn result in generalized slowing down of metabolic process characterized by broad clinical spectrum ranging from an asymptomatic or subclinical condition to fully manifested clinical condition. It is more common in females than males with middle age women more effected. The symptoms of hypothyroidism in middle age females are similar to ageing or menopause and it mislead to menopause. In infants one out of 5000 born without thyroid gland. It is more common than our perception and millions of people are currently suffering from hypothyroidism without knowing.

As far as the name of disease is concerned, no specific term is found for hypothyroidism in Ayurvedic classics. Though many diseases of current era do not mention in Ayurvedic texts, yet they can be successfully treated due to deep insight provided by the Ayurvedic principles. According to **Acharya Charak**, it is not necessary that every disease manifestation must have certain name, but it is more important to understand the possible pathogenesis of the disease in terms of involved factors like *Dosha, Dushya* etc. After knowing that, it can be successfully treated. The analysis of the symptomatology of hypothyroidism in the light of Ayurvedic principles show that the pathogenesis and manifestations of hypothyroidism occurs due to dysfunction of *Agni*.

It all starts with improper diet (heavy, cold, sweet and saturated fat containing food items) and sedentary lifestyle (lack of physical activity, sleeping after meals, sleeping during day time) which is now-a-day very common. It leads to aggravation of *Kapha*. The increased amount of *Kapha* impairs the *Jatharagni* with the formation of *Aamdosha*. As *Dhatvagni* depends on *Jatharagni bala*, so impairment of *Dhatvagni* takes place in due course of time. The effect of hypothyroidism is alteration in metabolic activity which, according to **Ayurveda**, is vitiation of *Dhatvagni*. This *Dhatvagni* vitiation causes improper formation of *Sapta dhatu* starting from *Rasa* to *Shukra*. It leads to improper nourishment to the body leading to symptoms of hypothyroidism along with swelling in neck described as *'Galgand'* in Ayurvedic texts.

So, there is a great need to find out a safe and effective remedy which not only relieve symptoms but also increase in sense of well-being leading to more acceptability and better compliance. Extensive research has been carried out all over the world in exploring new modes of treatment for hypothyroidism. It can be traced from rich, time-tested unsheathed treasure of knowledge of **Ayurveda**.

Ayurveda is a science of life with sole aim of providing health to the mankind. It has been able to maintain its glory and sustain its relevance beyond time due to the fact that it is practised on the laws of nature and not merely on tentative rules of medicine. It is the science of life, with a practical approach and scientific research in the field of life, provide us ground to reach the truth, to know the spheres and its limitations and finally to know its applied aspect. Both theoretical and practical knowledge led to new invention, discovery and achievements.

It can offer new dimensions towards understanding the aetiopathogenesis and successful management of hypothyroidism

Hypothyroidism is a disease with *Kapha Vata* predominance and *Pittakshaya*. In Hypothyroidism *Jatharagni Mandhya* leads to *Dhatvagni Mandhya*. Further hypothyroidism is a disease which may also be due to auto immunity. Looking the pathogenesis and complications of hypothyroidism, it requires a systemic and radical therapy for which Ayurveda may provide a ray of hope through *Panchakarma Chikitsa*.

The basic principle of **Ayurveda** is to augment the deficiency, to suppress the aggravation, reduce the increment of *Doshas* and also maintain the equilibrium of *Doshas* in healthy state. **Ayurveda** advocates two kinds of treatment measures, which represent the end-phase of all the treatment process, namely *Samshodhana* (Purificatory or eliminatory) and *Samshamana* (Pacificatory) of which the former is given the first place. *Doshas* once cured by pacification may circumstantially be provoked again, where as it can't ever do so, once it is totally expelled from the system by purification.

In Ayurveda, there is no direct mention of thyroid gland, but a disease by the name *Galgand*, characterized by neck swelling, is well known. The symptoms of *Galaganda* and hypothyroidism are vaguely similar. *Galgand* is explained in all the Ayurvedic texts.

HISTORICAL REVIEW

In **Charak Samhita,** *Galgand* explained in *Sutra Sthan* and *Chikitsa sthan* as:

यस्य श्लेष्मा प्रकुपितो गलबाह्येऽवतिष्ठते ।
शनैः संजनयेच्छोफं गलगण्डोऽस्य जायते ।। च. सू. 18/21

A swelling that is caused when a vitiated *Kapha* affects the throat from the outside and gradually produces swelling, is called *Galaganda*. **Acharya Sushrut** has defined *Galgand* in *Nidaan sthan*. The deranged & aggravated *Vata* in combination with the deranged and augmented *Kapha* and fat of the locality affects the two tendons of the neck and gradually give rise to a swelling about that part of the neck characterized by the specific symptoms of the deranged *Doshas* (*Vayu & Kapha*) and principles involved in the case. The swelling is called *Galagand*. As quoted by **Acharya Madhav**,

निबद्धः श्वयथुर्यस्य मुष्कवल्लम्बते गले।
महान् वा यदि वा ह्स्वो गलगण्डं तमादिशेत्।। मा.नि. 38/1

Bhav Prakash has given explanation of *Galgand* in *Chikitsa Sthan*. **Chakradatt** has defined *Galgand* in *Chikitsa Sthan*. Although, after mere knowledge of disorder pertaining the thyroid gland from view of modern system of medicines, one can't directly correlate this in **Ayurveda** as a whole disease yet signs and symptoms which we approach in day-to-day clinical practice can be seen in Ayurvedic texts.

INVOLVEMENT OF AGNI IN HYPOTHYROIDISM

Normalcy of all mechanisms of the body is totally dependent upon the normal functioning of *Agni*. According to Modern system of Medicine, metabolic activity of the body is controlled by thyroid hormone secretion and if we move our eyes towards **Ayurveda**, we will find that metabolic processes of the body are under the control of *Jatharagni*, *Bhutagni* and *Dhatvagni*, as quoted by **Charak**.

So, the cause of disease i.e. impaired metabolism can be compared with vitiation of *Agni* according to **Ayurveda**. If due to any etiological factor causing vitiation of *Agni*, whatsoever it may be, *Agni* gets vitiated resulting in start of pathological events which, eventually, leads to diseased condition of the body. This vitiation of *Agni* results in formation of *Ama Dosha* (undigested food). This *Ama Dosha* can be produced at three levels-

1.AT JATHARAGNI LEVEL - Due to improper digestion of food in *Amashaya* (because of hypo functioning of *Jatharagni*), products undergo some toxic changes called as *Ama*. According to modern science intestinal dys-biogenesis, infection, leaky gut are responsible for the development of immune dysregulation or autoimmunity which is the cause of the disease and can be correlated with *Ama*.

2.AT BHUTAGNI LEVEL - Physio-chemical aspect of digestion is dealt with *Bhutagnipaka*. Whenever *Ahara* (diet) is unprepared or uncooked, though at an early stage respective *Bhutagni* accept it and may digest but continuous supply of this *Nidana* (etiology) makes changes in *Bhutagni* also.

As far as thyroid physiology is concerned, iodine is nothing but *Bhutagni* only. Selective trapping of Iodide, transport, uptake by thyroid cells and organification- these all come under *Bhutagni Paka*. Intrathyroid and peripheral tissue deiodinase enzymes, thyro-peroxidase (TPO) and H_2O_2 can be considered as *Bhutagni Amsha* only and deficient iodine trapping or deficient iodine coupling or deficient enzymes, deiodinases are the causes of the disease according to modern medicine. Unless and until the internal factor is not vitiated fully, full-fledged pathogenesis cannot be possible.

3.AT DHATVAGNI LEVEL - *Ama* at *Dhatvagni* level can be considered to have two-fold origin:

- On the basis of exterior factor (when *Asthayi Poshkamsha* of *Dhatu* is in vitiated form)
- Due to interior factor –when tissue capacity to digest (*Dhatvagni*) even the balanced *Poshakamsha* (nutrients) is hampered.

Vagbhat has co-related *Jatharagni* to *Dhatvagni* carrying a suggestion that contributes moieties of itself to *Dhatus*. An increase in *Pachakagni* makes an increase of *Dhatus*, other *Agnis* and vice versa. Hence Due to improper functioning (Hypofunctioning) of *Pachakamsha* present in

Dhatus leads to states analogous to myxoedema resulting in *Dhatu Vriddhi*. Impaired *Dhatvagni* can be correlated with different chemical reactions like impaired glycogenolysis, impaired mitochondrial oxidation etc. in hypothyroidism.

STATUS OF AMA IN HYPOTHYROIDISM

स्रोतोरोधबलभ्रन्शगौरवानिलमूढताः ।
आलस्यापक्तिनिष्ठीवमलसङ्गारुचिक्लमाः ।। अ.ह.सू. 13/23-24

Clinical presentation of hypothyroidism includes, symptoms like lethargy, fatigue, weakness, heaviness in the body, sleepiness, hypochlorhydria, constipation, loss of appetite which denote presence of *Aamavastha* in the disease.

Looking in to clinical presentation of Hypothyroidism, involvement of *Tridosha* should be considered in which *Kapha Dosha* is main culprit associated with *Pitta Kshaya* and *Margavaranajanya Vata Vriddhi* can be considered.

Most of the symptoms of Hypothyroidism show *Kapha* dominance. Glycosaminoglycans deposition in the tissues can be considered as *Kapha Vargiya Dravya* which will cause obstruction in the channels and hence obstruction to the proper movement of *Vayu* producing *Margavaranajanya Vata Prakopa.* Impaired metabolism can be considered as *Pitta Dushti*.

Table: Involvement of Tridosha in Hypothyroidism

Sr.No.	Symptoms	*Dosha* involved	Reference
1.	Weight Gain	Kapha Vriddhi Pitta Kshaya	Ch.Su.17/56, A.H.Su.11/7 Ch. Su.20/17
2.	Puffiness of body parts	Kapha Vriddhi	Ch.Su.18, A.H.Su.12/53
3.	Loss of appetite	Kapha Vriddhi, Pitta Kshaya	A.H.Su.11/7, A.H.Su.11/16
4.	Dry and coarse skin	Vata Vriddhi, Pitta Kshaya	Ch. Su.20/17, Ch.Su.17/56
5.	Minimal or absent sweating	Pitta Kshaya	A.H.Su.12/52
6.	Anemia	Kapha Vriddhi, Pitta Kshaya, Vata Vriddhi	Ch. Su. 17/56
7.	Constipation	Vata Vraddhi	A.H.Su.11/6, Su.Su.15/18
8.	Hoarseness of voice	Kapha Vraddhi, Vata Vraddhi	Sharangdhar, Ch.Chi.16/24 Su.Su.15/18
9.	Generalized aches, Pain	Vata Vraddhi	Ch.Su.17/44
10.	Muscular cramps, Stiffness	Vata Vraddhi	Ch.Su.17/47, Su. Su.20/11
11.	Sluggishness	Kapha Vraddhi	Ch.Su.17/55

Also, some clinical conditions correlating with hypothyroidism described below include *Kapha* dominant conditions like *Kaphavritta UdanaVata*, *Kaphaja Pandu*, *Kaphaja Grahani* etc. Hence, the disease is *Tridoshaja* in nature.

Table: Involvement of Dhatu in Hypothyroidism

Sr. No.	Involved Dhatu	Symptoms	Reference
1.	Rasa	Weight Gain, Loss of appetite, lethargy, Generalized aches, Premature aging symptoms like hair loss etc. Cold intolerance, Puffiness, Anemia, Menstrual Disturbances, Infertility	Ch.Su.28/9-10; A.H.Su.11/7; Su. Su.15/32
2.	Rakta	Slow pulse rate, Dry and coarse Skin, Slowing of mental activity, Lethargy	Ch.Su.17/65; A.H.Su. 11/9; Su. Su.15/9
3.	Mamsa	Heavyness in the body, Muscle ache, Granthi, Galaganda	Su. Su. 15/14
4.	Meda	Tiredness, Sleepines, Sluggishness, Hyperlipidaemia, Dyspnea on exertion	Ch. Su. 28/13,14; Ch.Ni.4/47; A.H.11/11
5.	Asthi	Osteoporosis, Osteoarthritis	A.H.11/19
6.	Majja	Osteoporosis	A.H.11/19
7.	Shukra	Loss of libido, Infertility	Su. Su. 15/14

Because of wide ranging effects of thyroid hormone, Hypothyroidism can have profound detrimental effects on numerous organ systems.

Table: Involvement of Srotas in Hypothyroidism

S. N.	Involved Srotas	Symptoms	Reference
1.	Annavaha	Loss of appetite, Hypochlorhydria, Malabsorption	Ch. Vi. 5/8; Su. Sha. 9/64
2.	Rasavaha	Weight Gain, Loss of appetite, Heaviness in the body, lethargy, Generalized aches, Somnolence, Premature aging symptoms like hair loss etc. Cold intolerance, Puffiness, Anemia, Menstrual disturbances, Infertility	Ch.Su.28/9-10 Ch.Vi.5
3.	Raktavaha	Slow pulse rate, Dry and coarse skin, Slowing of mental activity, Lethargy, Anemia	Ch. Su. 24, Ch. Su. 28, Su. Sha. 9/17
4.	Mamsavaha	Oedema, Galaganda	Su. Sha. 9/18 Su.Su. 15/14
5.	Medovaha	Tiredness, Sleepiness, Sluggishness Hyperlipidemia, Dyspnea on exertion	Ch.Su. 28/13 Ch.Ni.4/47;
6.	Asthivaha	Osteoporosis, Osteoarthritis, Hair loss	Ch.SU.28/16 A.H.11/19
7.	Majjavaha	Osteoporosis	A.H.11/19

8.	Shukravaha	Loss of libido, Infertility	Su. Su. 15/14
9.	Purishvaha	Constipation	Ch. Vi 5
10.	Swedavaha	Sweating minimal/absent, Dry and coarse skin	Ch. Vi. 5
11.	Artavavaha	Loss of Libido, Infertility (secondary usually) Secondary amenorrhea	Su. Sha. 9

CLINICAL CONDITIONS SIMILAR TO HYPOTHYROIDISM

1. PITTA KSHAYA WITH KAPHA AND VATA VRIDDHI

Acharya Charak described a clinical condition in *Dosha Vikalpa Kalpana* presenting as *Pitta Kshaya* with *Kapha* and *Vata Vriddhi* which includes *Stambha* (Stiffness), *Shaitya* (cold intolerance), *Toda* (generalised aches), *Gaurava* (heaviness in the body), *Agni Mandya* (impaired metabolism), *Bhakta ashraddha* (Loss of appetite) shows resemblance with clinical presentation of hypothyroidism.

2. KAPHAVRITTA VATA

Symptoms quoted by **Acharya Charak** in *Kaphavritta Vata*, *Kaphavritta Udana*, *Kaphavritta Samana*, *Kaphavritta Vyana* conditions show similarity with clinical presentation of hypothyroidism to some extent.

3. KAPHAJA PANDU

Gaurava (heaviness in body), *Tandra* (sleepiness), *Panduta* (pallor), *Klama* (fatigue), *Shvasa* (dyspnea on exertion), *Aalasya* (lethargy),

Aruchi (loss of appetite), *Swara graha* (hoarseness of voice), *Ushnakamita* are the symptoms of *Kaphaja Pandu* which show similarity with hypothyroidism.

4. KAPHAJA GRAHANI

Purvarupa of *Grahani* like *Aalasya* (lethargy), *Balakshaya* (weakness), *Anna Vidaha*, *Sharira Gaurava* (Heaviness in body) and *Rupa* (symptoms) of *Kaphaja Grahani* like *Strishu Aharshanam* (loss of libido), *Akrashasyaapi Daurbalyam* can be correlated with clinical features of hypothyroidism. This condition denotes poor gut health which is responsible for suppression of thyroid hormones.

5. BAHUDOSHA LAKSHANA

Most of the symptoms of *Bahu Doshavastha* show clinical features similar with hypothyroidism.

NIDANA (ETIOLOGY)

Glancing at the nature of the disease, it can be concluded that *Dhatvagni Vikriti* (Hypo functioning) plays very important role in causing pathogenesis which in turn is caused by hyperfunctioning of *Jatharagni*. As the prime factor in causation of disease is *Agnimandya*, therefore, factors causing vitiation of *Agni* can be considered under *Nidana* factors of the disease.

1. Physiological factors affecting *Dhatvagni* like *Prakriti*, *Ritu*, *Bala*,

Age, Psychological factors when, tend to be abnormal, cause pathogenesis.

2. Under *Adhyatamika Hetus*, *Adibala Pravritta*, *Janmabala Pravritta* and *Dosha Bala Pravritta Hetus* help in causing diseased condition.

- In *Adibala Pravritjanya Vyadhi*, *Bijabhaga Dushti* takes place. According to modern, inheritance may be the cause (Congenital Hypothyroidism).
- Under *Janmabala Pravritta Vyadhis*, **Sushrut** has given examples of *Muka*, *Vamana*, *Jada* types. Here, *Jada* (*Mandabuddhi*) can be considered as Neonatal Hypothyroidism.
- Vitiation of *Sharira* as well as *Mansika Dhoshas* may be the causative factors considered under *Dosha Bala Pravritta Hetus*.

3. As we know that *Dhatu Parampara* (qualitative and quantitative production of *Dhatus*) is maintained by two factors.

- Intensity of *Agni*.
- Availability of the fuel (*Ahara Rasa*)

Therefore, anything affecting these two factors can be considered to cause disease. Excessive intake of water, erratic intake of food, *Vegavidharana* (suppression of urge), and day sleep etc. and psychological factors e.g. anxiety, fear, greed, anger and jealousy.

4. Non-gratification and dishonour of the desires of *Dauhrida* can lead

to the occurrence of disease. This can be interpreted as follows-

- According to **Sushrut**, development of fetus takes place in fourth month which is also a stage of *Dauhrida* in mother. If, at this stage, mother's desires are not fulfilled then it may lead to the birth of a paralyzed, hump-backed, crooked arms, lame, dwarfed, defective eyed child etc. This condition may be analysed according to modern parlance as a child of congenital hypothyroidism (cretinism) (i.e. stunting of body growth and retardation of mental development).
- According to modern science, thyroid is formed in 8th week and trapping of I_2 occurs from 12th week (4th month) which is again, a period of *Dauhrida* as per **Ayurveda**.

This may happen that non gratification of mother's desires at this stage may lead to deformity in particular organ functions. This hypothesis, however, needs further evaluation.

PURVARUPA (PRODROMAL SYMPTOMS)

Purvarupas are the caution lights to warn the patient and doctor about the pathogenesis happening in the body and makes us run towards exact diagnosis of the disease. In Hypothyroidism, it goes unnoticed for several years. Therefore, prodromal features are not mentioned in books.

RUPA (SYMPTOMS)

Rupa is a manifested stage of disease. It, on one hand, provides clue for the confirmed diagnosis and simultaneously, on the other hand, talks about severity and chronicity of the diseased condition. *Rupas* always appear after *Dosha-dushya-sammurcchna*. *Rupa* (symptomatology) of this disease as per **Ayurveda** is as follows-

1.ABNORMAL WEIGHT GAIN – It occurs due to imbalance between calorie intake and energy expenditure which, in hypothyroidism results due to disturbed metabolic processes. This can be considered as ***Dhatvagni*** Mandya (hypofunctioning) which causes Dhatuvraddhi .

2.PUFFY APPEARANCE OF BODY PARTS- Puffiness of face especially eyelids, hands and feet result due to accumulation of hydrophilic mucoproteins subcutaneously which may be categorized under *Kaphavargiya Dravya* as per **Ayurveda**. As *Kapha* is found in augmented state, due to its *Prithvi* and *Apa Mahabhuta* predominance, properties of heaviness and steadiness, this puffiness appears.

3.LOSS OF APPETITE – It may happen as a result of hypo functioning of *Jatharagni* which produces *Ama* and *Kapha* which further causes *Jatharagni* and *Dhatvagnimandya*.

4.DRY, COARSE SKIN / HAIR – *Rasa Dhatvagni Mandya* produces vitiated *Rasa Dhatu* which leads to improper nutrition to *Uttara Dhatu* i.e. *Rakta*, therefore leads to coarseness of skin & hair. Vitiated *Vata*

Dosha also causes dryness of skin. Moreover, *Twaka*, *Updhatu* of *Mamsa Dhatu*, gets affected because of vitiated *Mamsa Dhatu* & loses normalcy.

5.MINIMAL / ABSENT SWEATING – Physiologically, body temperature is controlled by *Pitta* because it loses excessive heat from the body in the form of *Sweda* (sweat). Its hypo functioning leads to above said manifestation.

6. ANAEMIA – In succession to *Dhatvagnimandya*, *Rasa Dhatu* get vitiated which is unable to nourish *Uttara* (next) *Dhatu*, *Rakta*. *Pandu* (Anaemia) has been described under *Rasa Dushtijanya Vikara* too.

7.CONSTIPATION –*Vayu Prakopa* results in *Gadhavarchastvam* (constipation) and aggravated *Kapha* (*Manda Guna*) may cause decrease in *Apa Karshani Gati* of *MahaSrotas* which leads to constipation.

8.HOARSENESS OF VOICE – Hoarseness of voice in hypothyroidism, mostly results either from mucinous deposits in vocal cords (intralaryngeal cause) or by external pressure on laryngeal nerve (extralaryngeal cause). According to **Sharangdhar**, hoarseness of voice arises from vitiated *Kapha* (*Manda Guna*).

9.GENERALISED ACHES AND PAIN – *Rasaja Vikara* arises from *Dhatvagnimandya* and aggravated *Vata Dosha* (increased *Toda*) may lead to causation of this symptom.

10.SLUGGISHNESS – In other words, *Shaithilaya*, *Alasya* (lazyness) results from vitiated *Rasa* and *Kapha*.

11.TIREDNESS – It results from aggravated *Vata* due to increased *Shrama*.

12.MENSTRUAL DISTURBANCES – Due to hypo functioning of *Agni*, *Rasa Vriddhi* result which is in *Asthayi* form. This vitiated *Dhatu* can't nourish *Updhatu Artava* and *Stanya* properly. Hence, menstruation caeses. Secondly, provocated *Doshas* causes *Artvavahasrotodushti* and obstruction of these *Srotas* results in *Anartva* (Secondary amenorrhoea).

13.COLD INTOLERANCE – Suppression of *Pitta Mandoshmata*, also propagation of *Shitaguna* of *Kapha* and *Rasa Dhatu* leads to *Shaitya*.

14. FORGETFULNESS – Vitiated *Kapha* may cause *Buddhimandya*. Also, *Manovaha Srotas* are affected by vitiated *Doshas*. All this makes a patient to be forgetful.

15.SLEEPINESS – Vitiated *Rasa* and *Kapha* induce sleepiness.

16.SLOW PULSE RATE – It may be due to *Manda Guna* of vitiated *Kapha*.

17.MUSCLE CRAMPS/STIFFNESS – It results due to over functioning of *Vayu*. Moreover, *Kandara* and *Snayu*, *Upadhatus* of *Rakta* and *Medodhatu* respectively, don't get proper nutrition which results in their improper function or it may be correlated with slow relaxation of muscles hence, stiffness ensues.

SAMPRAPTI (KRIYAKALA)

Acharya Sushrut has described *Shat Kriyakala* for the development of any disease which seems to be more logical and scientific in considering aetiopathogenesis of hypothyroidism according to **Ayurveda**. Here, a humble attempt is being made to describe pathogenesis of Hypothyroidism on the basis of *'Shat Kriyakala'*.

1. **Dosha Sanchayavastha:** In hypothyroidism, stress and other etiological factors stimulate brain and starts synthesizing or liberating certain biogenic amines. Due to various *Nidana* factors, *Tridosha* as well as *Agni* vitiation ensues, which results in augmentation and accumulation of *Kapha*.
2. **Second Kriya Kaal:** It is also known as *Kaal* of *Dosha Prakopavastha*. Aforesaid certain biogenic amines stimulate hypothalamus, pituitary, thyroid and adrenal medulla etc. Due to impairment of Agni, improper digestion of food results in production of *Ama Anna Rasa* which may further augment vitiated *Kapha*.
3. **Third Kriya Kaal:** This is a stage of *Dosha Prasaravastha*. Stimulation of above said glands induce secretion of releasing factors or hormones in the blood and biochemical alterations

get started. Vitiated *Rasa Dhatu* and *Rasagni Mandya* causes *Srotodusti*. Progression of the pathological events is ensued by *Uttarottara* (progressive) *Dhatvagnimandya* and *Uttarottara* vitiation of *Dhatus*. Moreover, circulation of *Ama Anna Rasa* may increase *Srotorodha*.

4. **Fourth Kriya Kaal**: This stage can be termed as *Sthanasamshraya*. Aforesaid, bio- chemical alterations start inducing an organopathological change in thyroid gland which depends upon tissue or cell susceptibility. Vitiated *Rasa* and augmented *Kapha* create *Dosha Dushya Sammurchna*.
5. **Fifth Kriya Kaal**: also called as *Vyaktavastha*. Organopathological changes happening in thyroid gland start developing their various signs and symptoms in different systems of the body. *Doshadushya Sammurchna*, if not treated, leads to manifestation of symptoms of disease.
6. **Sixth Kriya Kaal**: Progression of disease untreated with manifestation of complications results. E.g. Myxedema Coma, Myxedema madness.

AYURVEDIC PATHOGENESIS

Different *Aaharaja* (dietary), *Viharaja* (lifestyle) and *Manasika* (psychological) etiological factors will lead to *Tridosha* vitiation including dominance of *Kapha* associated *Pitta Dushti* and *Margavaranajanya Vata Prokopa*. This *Dosha* vitiation and

Agnimandyakara Nidana will cause vitiation of *Agni* and vitiation of *Annavaha Srotas.*

When *Jatharagni* gets impaired, on one hand, this *Jatharagnimandya* leads to formation of *Aama* (qualitative) which in turn causes *Rasavaha Srotodushti* and *Srotorodha.* while, on the other hand, its moieties which are distributed to *Dhatvagnis* get impaired disturbing status of *Dhatvagnis* too. Due to above pathological sequences, vitiated *Rasa Dhatu* is formed causing impairment of other *Dhatus* too *and Malarupi Kapha Vriddhi* will lead to *Srotolepa* causing again *Rasavaha Srotodushti.*

Thus, a chain of pathological events is started producing symptoms of *Rasa Dushti* like *Aruchi* (loss of appetite), *Gaurava* (Heaviness), *Tandra* (sleepiness), *Panduta* (pallor), *Srotorodha* (obstruction of channels) etc. Vitiated *Rasa Dhatu* will produce vitiated *Uttarottara Dhatu* with respective *Sroto Dushti* and thus a syndrome involving many organ systems will get developed.

TYPES OF GALGAND

According to **Acharya Sushrut**, three types of *Galgand*

- *Vataj Galgand*
- *Kaphaj Galgand*
- *Medoja Galgand*

Pittaj Galgand not described in any ayurvedic text.

SAMPRAPTI GHATAKA

- **Dosha**: *Kapha Vriddhi* associated with *Pitta Dushti* and *Margavaranajanya Vata Vriddhi*
- **Dushya**: *Rasa, Meda* predominantly
- **Agni**: *Jatharagni, Dhatvagni*
- **Ama**: *Jatharagni mandya Janita, Dhatvagnimandya Janita*
- **Srotas**: *Rasavaha Srotas,Medovaha Srotas* predominantly
- **Srotodusti**: *Sanga, Vimarga-gamana*
- **Adhisthana**: *Galpradesha* (Thyroid Gland)
- **Udbhavasthana**: *Amashaya*
- **Rogamarga**: *Bahya*
- **Vyaktisthana**: *Sharira*

Galgand is described in **Charak**, **Sushrut**, **Madhav Nidan**, **Bhav Prakash** and **Sharangdhar**.

SADHYATA - ASADHYATA

Prognosis, in case of adult hypothyroidism is good, if the ailment is started early (without complication). Patients generally lead to normal life after treatment. Once the therapy is started, it should be continued for long. According to **Ayurveda**, *Vyadhi* can be considered as *Krichhasadhaya*.

CHIKITSA (TREATMENT)

Health is like a vehicle which runs only on the balanced motion of four wheels viz. *Sharira*, *Indriya*, *Satva* and *Atma*. Any deterioration to above leads to diseased condition. To get rid of this deterioration, *Chikitsa* is essential.

In treatment of Hypothyroidism, by keeping the impairment of metabolism at base, we can treat patients fruitfully by acquiring *Agnivardhaka Chikitsa*. But an increase in *Pitta* need not always result in an increase of *Agni* digestive efficiency. It depends on *Amshamsha Kalpana* or *Vikalpa Samprapti*. In other words, it depends upon the nature and degree of increase of *Pachaka Pitta*. Capacity of digestion depends upon qualitative increase of *Ushna Guna* of *Pitta* whereas quantitative increase leads to increase in *Dravata* which results in *Agnimandya*. Therefore, drugs which increase digestive capacity of *Pitta* (quality of *Pitta*) can help in combating *Samprapti* of the disease.

SAMANYA CHIKITSA

According to **Yoga Ratnakar**

- Kanchnar Guggulu and Triphala Guggulu
- Nirgundi Tail, Gunja Tail
- Gandamala Kandan Rasa
- Pippali Churna
- Vradhi Vatika Vati and Arogyavardhini Vati

According to **Bhava Prakash**

- Kanchanar twak Kwath with Shunthi churna indicated in Galagand Gandamala Apachi Granthi Arbud Adhikar
- Chakramarda taila, Amritadi taila, Jalkumbhi Bhasma with Saindhava lavana and Pippali

According to **Chakradatt**

- Nimb tail Nasya indicated in Galagand Gandamala Apachi Granthi Arbud Adhikar
- Jalkumbhi Bhasma with Gomutra.

- $$$ -

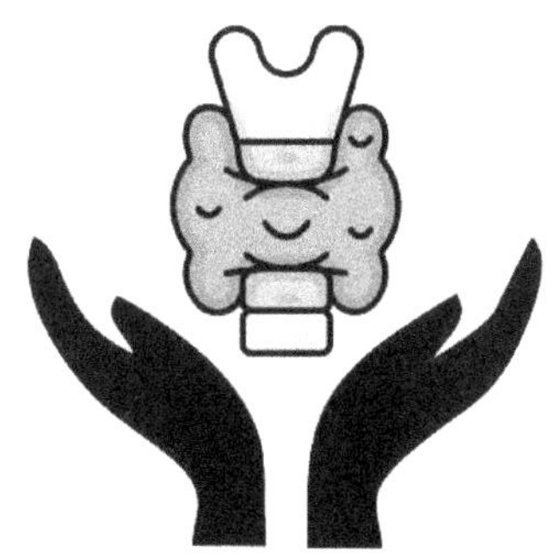

Thyroid Anatomy

Dr. Tina Singhal

The word Thyroid is derived from Greek word *'Thyros'* which means Shield and *'Eidos'* means form which denotes that this gland has been named after it Shield like appearance. Thyroid gland regulates the all-body functions, including metabolic, Respiratory, Cardiovascular, Digestive, Nervous & Reproductive systems either directly or indirectly. Thyroid is two lobed glands situated at the root of the neck on either side of the Trachea and this gland secretes three hormones like Tetra-iodothyronine T_4 (thyroxine), Tri-iodothyronine T_3, Calcitonin. T_4 & T_3 both are iodine containing derivatives of amino acid tyrosine. T_4 forms about 90% of the total secretion and T_3 is only 9-10% but the potency of T_3 is 4 times more than that of T_4. Iodine and Tyrosine are essential for the formation of thyroid hormones and both are absorbed from GI tract.

Disease of the Thyroid predominantly effect females and are more common occurring in about 5% of the population. Sign & Symptoms of hypothyroidism i.e. swelling of the face, Bagginess under the eyes, non-pitting type edema, Atherosclerosis and other general features of hypothyroidism i.e. Anemia, Fatigue & Muscle sluggishness, Extreme Somnolence with sleeping, Menorrhagia (commonly) but Amenorrhea & oligomenorrhea may be occur, Increase body weight, Constipation, Mental sluggishness, Depressed Hair Growth and cold intolerance etc. Hypothyroidism occurs when the thyroid is hypoactive and does not produce enough thyroid hormones. Goiter is produced by the inadequate secretion of thyroid hormones, resulting in positive feedback of a pituitary hormone, TSH on the thyroid gland that ultimately enlarges.

ANATOMY

Normal adult thyroid gland is the largest endocrine gland in the body having a tremendous capacity to get further enlarged. It weighs about 20 gm and is found larger in females during menstruation and pregnancy. The thyroid gland, located in the anterior neck just below the cricoid cartilage. Gland, situated in lower neck at the levels of C_5, C_6, C_7 & T_1 vertebra, consists of two lobes connected by isthmus that crosses the front of 2nd and 3rd tracheal rings. Shape of the gland is just like a large plum half cut (vertically).

KEY FEATURES OF THE THYROID GLAND

- **Two lobes:** The right and left lobes are the main parts of the gland.
- **Isthmus:** The isthmus is the connecting bridge between the two lobes.
- **Pyramidal lobe:** A small, upward extension of the isthmus may be present in some individuals.
- **Follicles:** The functional units of the thyroid gland are called follicles. These are tiny spheres lined with cells that produce thyroid hormones.
- **Blood vessels:** The thyroid gland has a rich blood supply, ensuring efficient delivery of hormones into the bloodstream.
- **Nerves:** The thyroid gland is innervated by both sympathetic and parasympathetic nerves, which regulate its function.

LOCATION

The thyroid gland is situated in the anterior part of neck, anterior to the trachea and larynx. It is typically located between the fifth cervical vertebra and the first thoracic vertebra.

HISTOLOGY

Thyroid gland is composed of vesicles called as follicles or acini surrounded by capillary network. Follicle walls are composed of cuboidal epithelium. Lumen is filled with proteinaceous colloid which contains a protein peculiar to thyroid, thyroglobulin, in which peptide sequence T_3 & T_4 are synthesized and stored. Gland also contains a smaller second population of cells i.e., parafollicular cells (C cells) secrete the hormone calcitonin, which is released in response to hypercalcemia and lowers serum Ca levels.

KEY HISTOLOGICAL FEATURES

1. THYROID FOLLICLES

- These are the structural and functional units of the thyroid gland.
- They are spherical structures lined by a single layer of cuboidal epithelial cells called follicular cells.
- The lumen of each follicle is filled with a viscous, protein-rich fluid called colloid.

2. FOLLICULAR CELLS

- These cells are responsible for synthesizing and secreting thyroid hormones (T3 and T4).
- They actively transport iodine from the bloodstream into the colloid.
- Within the colloid, they synthesize the thyroid hormone precursor, thyroglobulin.
- They also reabsorb thyroglobulin from the colloid and cleave it to release T3 and T4 into the bloodstream.

3. COLLOID

- This is the gel-like material that fills the lumen of the follicles.
- It primarily consists of thyroglobulin, a large glycoprotein that serves as a storage form for thyroid hormones.
- It also contains iodine, which is essential for thyroid hormone synthesis.

4. PARAFOLLICULAR CELLS (C CELLS)

- These are specialized cells located between the follicular cells.
- They are responsible for producing and secreting calcitonin, a hormone that helps regulate blood calcium levels.

BLOOD SUPPLY

The thyroid gland has an exceptionally rich blood supply, ensuring efficient delivery of hormones into the bloodstream.

- **Superior Thyroid Artery:** This branch of the external carotid artery supplies the superior part of the gland.
- **Inferior Thyroid Artery:** This branch of the thyrocervical trunk supplies the inferior part of the gland.
- **Thyroid Ima Artery:** This variable artery may arise from the brachiocephalic trunk or the aortic arch and contributes to the blood supply of the gland.

VENOUS DRAINAGE

Venous blood from the thyroid gland is primarily drained by:

- **Superior Thyroid Vein:** This drains into the internal jugular vein.
- **Middle Thyroid Vein:** This drains into the internal jugular vein.
- **Inferior Thyroid Vein:** This drains into the left brachiocephalic vein.

NERVE SUPPLY

The thyroid gland receives both sympathetic and parasympathetic innervation:

- **Sympathetic Innervation:** This originates from the cervical ganglia of the sympathetic trunk and primarily regulates blood flow to the gland.
- **Parasympathetic Innervation:** This originates from the vagus nerve and may influence hormone secretion.

FUNCTION OF THYROID GLAND

The thyroid gland is a vital part of the endocrine system and plays a crucial role in regulating various bodily functions through hormone production. Here's a summary of its functions:

1. Hormone Production: It produces two main hormones, thyroxine (T_4) and triiodothyronine (T_3), which are essential for normal metabolism, growth, and development.

2. Metabolic Regulation: T_3 and T_4 hormones increase the basal metabolic rate, influencing the number of calories the body needs to function at rest.

3. Calcium and Bone Metabolism: The thyroid also produces calcitonin, which helps regulate calcium and phosphate levels in the blood.

4. Hormone Synthesis: The thyroid gland synthesizes hormones by utilizing iodine from the diet. The primary hormones produced are thyroxine (T_4) and triiodothyronine (T_3), which regulate the body's metabolic processes.

5. Metabolic Effects: T_3 and T_4 hormones increase the basal metabolic rate, which is the rate at which the body uses energy while at rest. They influence metabolism, growth, and development, including the metabolism of carbohydrates and fats.

6. Regulation of Body Functions: Thyroid hormones play a role in regulating various body functions such as breathing, heart rate, central and peripheral nervous systems, body weight, muscle strength, menstrual cycles, body temperature, and cholesterol levels.

7. Calcitonin: Besides T_3 and T_4, the thyroid gland also produces calcitonin, which helps in calcium and bone metabolism. It regulates calcium levels in the blood and bone turnover.

8. Feedback Mechanism: The production of thyroid hormones is regulated by a feedback mechanism involving the hypothalamus and the pituitary gland. The pituitary gland releases thyroid-stimulating hormone (TSH), which stimulates the thyroid to produce T_3 and T_4.

9. Impact on Mood and Energy: Thyroid hormones can affect mood and energy levels. Imbalances in these hormones can lead to conditions such as depression or anxiety.

10. Influence on Fertility: Thyroid hormones are also important for reproductive health. They can influence fertility, ovulation, and menstruation.

11. Disease Conditions: Conditions such as Hashimoto's thyroiditis and Graves' disease can disrupt the normal function of the thyroid, leading to hypothyroidism or hyperthyroidism, respectively. Maintaining a healthy thyroid gland is essential for overall well-being, as it influences so many aspects of human health. If you suspect any issues with your thyroid function, it's important to consult with a healthcare provider for proper diagnosis and treatment.

- $$$ -

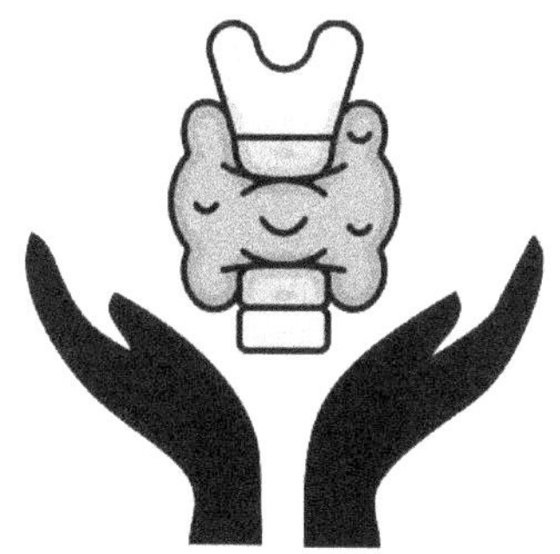

HYPOTHYROIDISM: A BRIEF OVERVIEW

Dr. Pratima Yadav, Dr Ajay Kumar

Hypothyroidism is a clinical syndrome which results from deficiency of thyroid hormones. **Cretinism** is termed when Hypothyroidism ages from birth and results in developmental abnormalities. **Myxedema** is defined as severe Hypothyroidism in which there is accumulation of hydrophilic mucopolysaccharides in dermis and other tissues leading to thickness of the facial features and doughy indurations of the skin.

PREVALENCE

- Congenital Hypothyroidism is common in India, the disease occurring 1 in 2640 neonates when compared with worldwide average value of 1 in 3800 subjects.
- Adult Hypothyroidism-3.9%
- Subclinical Hypothyroidism-9.4 %

- Female-11.4% and male-6.2
- Race: NHANES 1999-2002 reported that the prevalence of Hypothyroidism (including subclinical) was higher in whites (5.1%) and Mexican Americans than in African Americans (1.7%). African Americans tend to have lower TSH values.

ETIOLOGY OF HYPOTHYROIDISM

Hypothyroidism is a prevalent endocrine disorder characterized by the **thyroid gland's insufficient production of thyroid hormones**. The condition affects women more frequently than men, with a female-to-male ratio of 6:1.

The etiology of hypothyroidism varies depending on the geographical prevalence of iodine deficiency. In regions with **adequate iodine intake**, the most common causes are:

- **Autoimmune thyroiditis (Hashimoto's thyroiditis):** This condition involves the immune system attacking the thyroid gland, leading to inflammation and destruction of thyroid tissue.
- **Iatrogenic hypothyroidism:** This form of hypothyroidism arises as a consequence of medical interventions, primarily:
- **Radioactive iodine therapy:** This treatment, frequently employed for hyperthyroidism, can inadvertently result in hypothyroidism.

- **Surgical thyroidectomy:** Surgical removal of the thyroid gland, performed for various thyroid conditions, inevitably leads to hypothyroidism.

Less common causes of hypothyroidism include:

- **Secondary hypothyroidism:** This occurs when the pituitary gland, responsible for stimulating thyroid hormone production, fails to produce sufficient **thyroid-stimulating hormone (TSH)**.
- **Transient thyroiditis:** Certain types of thyroiditis, such as subacute or postpartum thyroiditis, can cause temporary hypothyroidism.
- **Drug-induced hypothyroidism:** Medications like amiodarone, commonly prescribed for cardiac arrhythmias, can interfere with thyroid hormone synthesis and lead to hypothyroidism.
- **Dyshormonogenesis:** This rare condition encompasses a group of inherited disorders that impair the thyroid gland's ability to synthesize thyroid hormones effectively.

CLINICAL MANIFESTATIONS

The clinical presentation of hypothyroidism hinges on the **duration and severity of thyroid hormone deficiency**. The gradual onset of hypothyroidism, typically spanning months or years, allows the body to adapt to the hormonal deficit, resulting in subtle and insidious symptom development.

Hypothyroidism often manifests with **subtle, nonspecific symptoms** that gradually emerge over time. Recognizing these symptoms is crucial for timely diagnosis and management. Common symptoms include:

- **Fatigue:** A persistent feeling of tiredness and lack of energy, often interfering with daily activities.
- **Weight gain:** Unexplained weight gain despite normal dietary intake and physical activity.
- **Cold intolerance:** Increased sensitivity to cold temperatures, feeling cold even in mildly cool environments.
- **Dry skin:** Skin becomes rough, dry, and flaky due to decreased sweat and oil production.
- **Constipation:** Infrequent bowel movements and difficulty passing stools.
- **Depression:** Persistent feelings of sadness, hopelessness, and loss of interest in activities.
- **Impaired memory:** Difficulty in remembering things and concentrating.
- **Hoarseness:** A change in voice quality, becoming raspy or husky.
- **Hair loss:** Thinning of hair on the scalp and other body areas.

Physical examination findings that may indicate hypothyroidism include:

- **Bradycardia:** Slow heart rate, often below 60 beats per minute.
- **Hypothermia:** Low body temperature, typically below 98.6°F (37°C).
- **Delayed relaxation of deep tendon reflexes:** Sluggish reflexes, particularly noticeable in the ankle and knee jerks.
- **Dry, coarse skin:** Skin texture becomes rough and thickened due to decreased moisture.
- **Thinning of the eyebrows:** Loss of the outer third of the eyebrows, a characteristic sign of hypothyroidism.
- **Myxedema** (Nonpitting edema)**:** This characteristic finding involves the accumulation of glycosaminoglycans in the skin and subcutaneous tissues, leading to a puffy appearance, particularly around the eyes, hands, and feet.

DIAGNOSIS OF HYPOTHYROIDISM

Diagnosing hypothyroidism hinges on a combination of clinical symptoms and laboratory tests. The most reliable laboratory test is the **thyroid-stimulating hormone (TSH) test**, which measures the level of TSH produced by the pituitary gland. **Elevated TSH levels** indicate that the pituitary gland is overworking to stimulate the thyroid gland, a hallmark of hypothyroidism. While T3, or triiodothyronine, is another thyroid hormone, its measurement is not routinely recommended for hypothyroidism diagnosis. T3 levels may remain within the normal range in early or mild hypothyroidism, making it a less reliable marker.

The cornerstone of hypothyroidism diagnosis is **laboratory** assessment of **thyroid function**. The primary tests include:

- **TSH level:** TSH is the most sensitive indicator of hypothyroidism. In primary hypothyroidism, the TSH level is markedly **elevated**, reflecting the pituitary gland's attempt to stimulate the underactive thyroid gland.
- **Free Thyroxine (FT4):** Measures the level of unbound thyroxine (T4), the active form of thyroid hormone.
- **Total Thyroxine (T4):** Measures the total amount of T4 in the blood, including both bound and unbound forms.
- **Triiodothyronine (T3):** The active form of the hormone.

Additional laboratory tests that aid in diagnosing hypothyroidism include:

- **Thyroid Peroxidase Antibodies (TPOAb):** Detects antibodies against thyroid peroxidase, an enzyme involved in thyroid hormone production. Presence of these antibodies suggests autoimmune thyroiditis.
- **Thyroglobulin (TG):** A protein that is sometimes measured in blood tests.
- **Thyroglobulin Antibodies (TgAb):** Detects antibodies against

thyroglobulin, a protein produced by the thyroid gland. Presence of these antibodies also points towards autoimmune thyroiditis.

- **Thyroid-stimulating immunoglobulin (TSI):** An antibody that is sometimes measured in blood tests.
- **TSH Receptor-Stimulating Antibodies:** An antibody that is used to diagnose Graves' disease, an autoimmune condition that leads to hyperthyroidism.

MANAGEMENT OF HYPOTHYROIDISM

The cornerstone of hypothyroidism treatment is lifelong **thyroid hormone replacement therapy**. The most commonly prescribed medication is **levothyroxine**, a synthetic form of T4. It is administered orally once daily, typically in the morning before breakfast. The **dosage of levothyroxine is individualized** based on the patient's TSH levels and clinical response. Regular monitoring of TSH levels is crucial to ensure optimal dosage and symptom control.

Key aspects of levothyroxine therapy include:

- **Dose titration:** The optimal levothyroxine dose varies among individuals and is determined by monitoring TSH levels. The goal is to maintain TSH within the reference range, typically requiring a T4 level in the upper reference range.
- **Monitoring:** Regular monitoring of TSH levels is essential to ensure appropriate dose adjustments and maintain euthyroidism.

Factors influencing levothyroxine requirements:

- **Age:** Elderly patients may require lower doses of levothyroxine.
- **Comorbid conditions:** Certain medical conditions, such as heart disease, may necessitate cautious dose adjustments.
- **Concomitant medications:** Certain drugs, such as phenytoin, ferrous sulfate, and rifampicin, can interfere with levothyroxine absorption or metabolism.
- **Pregnancy:** Levothyroxine requirements often increase during pregnancy due to hormonal changes.

COMPLICATIONS OF HYPOTHYROIDISM

MYXEDEMA COMA

This rare but life-threatening complication of hypothyroidism represents a **medical emergency**. Myxedema coma typically occurs in elderly individuals with long-standing, severe hypothyroidism who experience a precipitating event, such as infection, cold exposure, or certain medications.

Hallmarks of Myxedema coma include:

- Depressed consciousness, ranging from confusion to coma
- Hypothermia (low body temperature)
- Hypoventilation (slowed breathing)
- Hypotension (low blood pressure)

- Hyponatremia (low sodium levels)

Myxedema coma carries a high mortality rate, emphasizing the importance of prompt recognition and aggressive treatment. Treatment involves:

- **Supportive Care:** Maintaining airway, breathing, and circulation is paramount.
- **Intravenous Thyroid Hormone Replacement:** Intravenous levothyroxine is administered to rapidly restore thyroid hormone levels.
- **Management of Associated Complications:** Addressing hypothermia, hyponatremia, and other metabolic derangements is crucial.

SUBCLINICAL HYPOTHYROIDISM

This condition, characterized by an **elevated TSH level with normal T3 and T4 levels**, represents a milder form of hypothyroidism. While subclinical hypothyroidism is often asymptomatic, it can progress to overt hypothyroidism over time. Individuals with subclinical hypothyroidism, particularly those with TSH levels above 10 mU/L or positive antithyroid peroxidase antibodies, should be monitored closely and considered for levothyroxine therapy to prevent progression and potential complications.

COMPLICATIONS OF UNTREATED HYPOTHYROIDISM

Failure to treat hypothyroidism can result in serious complications. These complications include:

- **Heart disease:** Hypothyroidism can contribute to heart disease by increasing cholesterol levels and impairing heart function. This can lead to atherosclerosis, coronary artery disease, and heart failure.
- **Infertility:** Hypothyroidism can disrupt ovulation and make it difficult to conceive. It can also increase the risk of miscarriage and preterm labor.
- **Birth defects:** Untreated hypothyroidism during pregnancy can harm fetal development and lead to birth defects, including intellectual disability and developmental delays.
- **Myxedema coma:** A rare but life-threatening complication characterized by severe hypothermia, altered mental status, and respiratory failure.

THE GUT-THYROID-IMMUNE CONNECTION

The gut is a hollow tube that passes from the mouth to the anus. Anything that goes in the mouth and isn't digested will pass right out the other end.

IMPORTANT FUNCTIONS OF THE GUT

- To prevent foreign substances from entering the body.
- To host 70% of the immune tissue in the body. This portion of the immune system is collectively referred to as GALT, or gut-associated lymphoid tissue. The GALT comprises several types of lymphoid tissues that store immune cells, such as T & B lymphocytes, that carry out attacks and produce antibodies against antigens, molecules recognized by the immune system as potential threats.

Problems occur when either of these protective functions of the gut are compromised. When the intestinal barrier becomes permeable (i.e. **leaky gut syndrome**), large protein molecules escape into the bloodstream. Since these proteins don't belong outside of the gut, the body mounts an immune response and attacks them. Studies show that these attacks play a role in the development of autoimmune diseases like Hashimoto's. Thyroid hormones strongly influence the tight junctions in the stomach and small intestine. These tight junctions are closely associated areas of two cells whose membranes join together to form the impermeable barrier of the gut. T_3 and T_4 have been shown to protect gut mucosal lining from stress induced ulcer formation. In another study, endoscopic examination of gastric ulcers found low T_3, low T_4 and abnormal levels of reverse T_3.

THE GUT-BACTERIA-THYROID CONNECTION

One little known role of the gut bacteria is to assist in converting inactive T_4 into the active form of thyroid hormone, T_3. About 20 percent of T_4 is converted to T_3 in the GI tract, in the forms of T_3 sulfate (T_3S) and triidothyroacetic acid (T_3AC). The conversion of T_3S and T_3AC into active T_3 requires an enzyme called intestinal sulfates. This enzyme comes from healthy gut bacteria. Intestinal dysbiosis, an imbalance between pathogenic and beneficial bacteria in the gut, significantly reduces the conversion of T_3S and T_3AC to T_3. This is one reason why people with poor gut function may have thyroid symptoms but normal lab results.

Inflammation in the gut also reduces T_3 by raising cortisol. Cortisol decreases active T_3 levels while increasing levels of inactive T_3. Studies have also shown that cell walls of intestinal bacteria, called lipopolysaccharides (LPS), negatively affect thyroid metabolism in several ways.

OTHER GUT-THYROID CONNECTIONS

- Hypochlorhydria, or low stomach acid, increases intestinal permeability, inflammation and infection Studies shown that a strong association between atrophic body gastritis, a condition related to hypochlorhydria, and autoimmune thyroid disease.

- Constipation can impair hormone clearance and cause elevations in estrogen, which in turn raises thyroid-binding globulin (TBG) levels and decreases the amount of free thyroid hormones available to the body. On the other hand, low thyroid function slows transit time, causing constipation and increasing inflammation, infections and malabsorption.
- Finally, a sluggish gall bladder interferes with proper liver detoxification and prevents hormones from being cleared from the body and Hypothyroidism impairs GB function by reducing bile flow.

GASTROINTESTINAL DYSBIOSIS & MALABSORPTION

When we don't have enough good bacteria present, the food we eat doesn't get broken down enough, and we lose out on the available nutrients in the food. Second, the undigested food causes the lining of the intestinal tract to become inflamed as it passes through. Over time, repeated episodes of inflammation cause the intestinal lining to become more porous, thereby allowing bigger particles of food and waste product to absorb through the intestinal wall and into the bloodstream. When this happens, your immune system is activated, surrounds, engulfs, and neutralizes the food particles. As you repeatedly eat these same foods, your immune system will begin to consistently attack them, developing into what we refer to as low grade food allergies or food sensitivities. This is a very important concept, since repeated activation of the immune system is what ultimately creates the environment for autoimmune disorders to begin. In this way, autoimmunity get developed due to poor gut health and become cause for Hypothyroidism.

In Hashimoto's thyroiditis, there is a marked lymphocytic infiltration of the thyroid with germinal center formation, atrophy of the thyroid follicles accompanied by oxyphil metaplasia, absence of colloid, and mild to moderate fibrosis. In atrophic thyroiditis, the fibrosis is much more extensive, lymphocyte infiltration is less pronounced, and thyroid follicles are almost completely absent. Atrophic thyroiditis likely represents the end stage of Hashimoto's thyroiditis rather than a distinct disorder.

The thyroid lymphocytic infiltrate in autoimmune Hypothyroidism is composed of activated CD4+ and CD8+ T cells, as well as B cells. Thyroid cell destruction is primarily mediated by the CD8+ cytotoxic T cells, which destroy their targets by either perforin-induced cell necrosis or granzyme B–induced apoptosis.

In addition, local T cell production of cytokines, such as tumor necrosis factor (TNF), IL-1, and interferon γ (IFN- γ), may render thyroid cells more susceptible to apoptosis mediated by death receptors, such as Fas, which are activated by their respective ligands on T cells. These cytokines also impair thyroid cell function directly and induce the expression of other proinflammatory molecules by the thyroid cells themselves, such as cytokines, HLA class I and class II molecules, adhesion molecules, CD40, and nitric oxide. Administration of high concentrations of cytokines for therapeutic purposes (especially IFN-γ) is associated with increased autoimmune thyroid disease, possibly through mechanisms.

MUCILAGINOUS OEDEMA

One important event in the pathogenesis of Hypothyroidism is deposition of hyaluronic acid i.e. mucopolysaccharides in the tissues and skin which leads to mucilaginous oedema. Deficiency of thyroid hormones inhibit the degradation of hyaluronic acid leading to its deposition.

MUCOPOLYSACCHARIDES

- These are long unbranched polysaccharides consisting of repeating disaccharides.
- Hyaluronan (also called hyaluronic acid or hyaluronate) is an anionic, no sulphated glycosaminoglycan distributed widely throughout connective, epithelial, and neural tissues. It is unique among glycosaminoglycans in that it is no sulfated, forms in the plasma membrane instead of the Golgi, and can be very large, with its molecular weight often reaching the millions.

- One of the chief components of the extracellular matrix, hyaluronan contributes significantly to cell proliferation and migration, and may also be involved in the progression of some malignant tumors.
- Hyaluronan is a major component of the synovial fluid, and was found to increase the viscosity of the fluid.
- Hyaluronan is an important component of articular cartilage, where it is present as a coat around each cell (chondrocyte).
- Hyaluronan is also a major component of skin, where it is involved in tissue repair. When skin is exposed to excessive UVB rays, it becomes inflamed (sunburn) and the cells in the dermis stop producing as much hyaluronan, and increase the rate of its degradation. Hyaluronan degradation products also accumulate in the skin after UV exposure.

- $$$ -

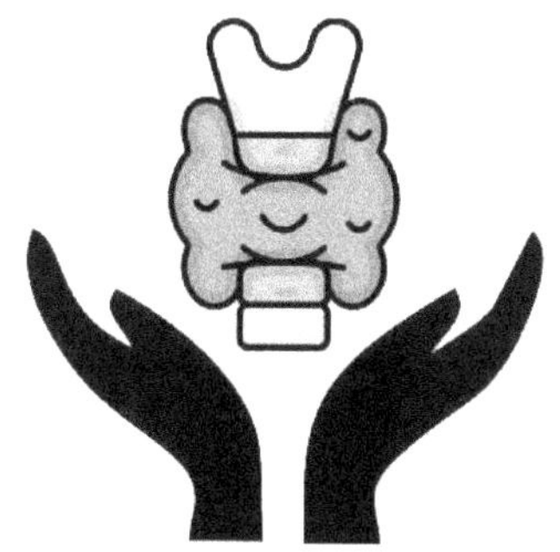

HYPERTHYROIDISM: BRIEF REVIEW

Dr Ajay Kumar, Dr. Pratima Yadav

Ayurveda categorizes hyperthyroidism as *Bhasmak Roga*, wherein the metabolic rate is remarkably elevated because of disturbed *Tridoshas*, with a decline in *Kapha Dosha* and an escalation in *Vata* and *Pitta Dosha*. This situation can be addressed through medications and treatments that calm the heightened *Pitta Dosha*. Nevertheless, hyperthyroidism is a state of hypermetabolism in the body resulting from excessive thyroid hormone production. it can be compared to *Atyagni, Tikshnagni*, or *Bhasmaka Roga*. Both *Bhasmaka Roga* and Hyperthyroidism, *Pitta Prakopa* (aggravation) play crucial role in the pathogenesis and symptomatology of both conditions. The two thyroid hormones, Tri-iodothyronine (T_3) and Thyroxine (T_4), function as *Pitta* within the body. An increase in these hormone levels results in accelerated digestion of food and subsequently, the depletion of *Dhatu* (tissues). If the patient withdraws from food, this elevation will enhance the *Jatharagni*, leading to the depletion of tissues and the onset of cachexia.

SYMPTOMS OF HYPERTHYROIDISM

Hyperthyroidism, also known as an overactive thyroid, occurs when thyroid gland produces too much of the thyroid hormone. This excess hormone can cause a wide range of symptoms that affect various bodily functions. Here are some common symptoms of hyperthyroidism:

- **Nervousness, anxiety, and irritability:** You might feel on edge, restless, or easily agitated.
- **Increased heart rate (tachycardia) and/or heart palpitations:** Your heart may beat faster than normal, and you might feel like it's fluttering or pounding in your chest.
- **Tremors, usually in the hands and fingers:** You might experience shaking or trembling, especially in your hands.
- **Weight loss despite a regular or increased appetite:** You might lose weight even though you're eating normally or even more than usual.
- **Increased sweating and sensitivity to warm temperatures:** You might sweat more than usual, even in cool temperatures. You might also feel uncomfortable in warm environments.

- **Fatigue and weakness:** You might feel tired all the time, even after getting enough sleep.
- **Difficulty sleeping (insomnia):** You might have trouble falling asleep or staying asleep.
- **Changes in menstrual periods:** Your periods might become lighter, shorter, or less frequent.
- **Enlargement of the thyroid gland (goiter)**: You might notice a swelling in your neck.
- **Swelling or bulging of the eyes (thyroid eye disease):** Your eyes might appear to be bulging or protruding.
- **Loose stools or diarrhea:** You might experience more frequent bowel movements that are loose or watery.
- **Heat intolerance**: You might feel uncomfortable in warm temperatures and prefer cooler environments.
- **Muscle weakness:** You might experience weakness or fatigue in your muscles.
- **Hair loss or thinning hair:** You might notice hair loss or thinning hair, especially on your scalp.
- **Skin changes:** Your skin might become thinner, more oily, or more sensitive.
- **Emotional changes:** You might experience mood swings, irritability, or anxiety.

- **Changes in appetite:** You might experience an increased or decreased appetite.
- **Changes in libido:** You might experience a decreased sex drive.

It's important to note that not everyone with hyperthyroidism will experience all of these symptoms, and the severity of symptoms can vary from person to person.

DIAGNOSIS OF HYPERTHYROIDISM

A blood test serves as a method to confirm the condition. TSH levels will be low, but levels of thyroid hormones will also be elevated. Elevated free thyroxine and free triiodothyronine levels indicate hyperthyroidism. Consequently, a thyroid scan may sometimes be necessary. Thyrotoxicosis is almost always caused by hyperthyroidism, but it can sometimes be caused by other conditions, such as thyroiditis or taking too much thyroid hormone.

The following methods can be used to diagnose thyrotoxicosis:

1) **Thyroid function tests (TFTs):** These measure blood levels of the thyroid hormones **triiodothyronine (T3)** and **thyroxine (T4)**. Most people with thyrotoxicosis have elevated T3 and T4.
    a) In **T3 toxicosis**, T4 is normal but T3 is elevated. This occurs in about 5% of patients.
    b) In primary thyrotoxicosis, serum thyroid-stimulating hormone (TSH) is undetectable.

   c) TFTs must be interpreted carefully during **pregnancy**, because pregnancy increases thyroid-binding globulin, which leads to higher total T3 and T4, while TSH reference ranges are lower. A **fully suppressed TSH with elevated free hormone levels indicates thyrotoxicosis** in pregnant patients.

2) **Antibody tests:** Elevated **TSH receptor antibodies (TRAb)** are found in 80–95% of patients with **Graves' disease**. Other thyroid antibodies are not specific for any particular thyroid condition.

3) **Imaging studies:**

   a) **99mTechnetium scintigraphy** can be used to determine the pattern of isotope uptake by the thyroid gland, which can help to determine the cause of thyrotoxicosis:

      i) **Graves' disease:** diffuse uptake

      ii) **Multinodular goitre:** low, patchy uptake within the nodules

      iii) **Toxic adenoma:** a hot spot is seen in the toxic adenoma, with no uptake in the dormant gland tissue

      iv) **Low-uptake thyrotoxicosis:** usually caused by transient thyroiditis. Rarely caused by factitious thyrotoxicosis due to taking thyroxine

b) **Thyroid scintigraphy** should be performed if a patient has a nodular thyroid and low serum TSH to confirm the presence of a hot nodule. If TSH is normal, scintigraphy is not routinely used to investigate thyroid nodules.

c) **Ultrasound** can be used to distinguish between generalized and localized thyroid swelling if thyroid function is normal.

   i) **Graves' disease and Hashimoto's thyroiditis** cause diffuse hypoechogenicity on ultrasound.

   ii) **Graves' disease** also causes increased thyroid blood flow on Doppler ultrasound.

d) **Ultrasound** can also be used to determine the size and number of thyroid nodules and whether nodules are solid or cystic. It is not reliable for distinguishing between benign and malignant nodules. However, features that suggest malignancy include hypervascularity, microcalcification, and irregular, infiltrative margins. A purely cystic nodule or a spongiform appearance suggest a benign etiology.

4) **Fine needle aspiration cytology:** This is recommended for most thyroid nodules that are larger than 1 cm in diameter. Smaller nodules can be observed with interval ultrasound scans if they have benign cytology and a reassuring ultrasound appearance.

CAUSES

Hyperthyroidism, or an overactive thyroid, can be caused by several factors that lead to excessive thyroid hormone production:

- **Graves' Disease:** This is the most common cause of hyperthyroidism. It's an autoimmune disorder where your immune system mistakenly attacks the thyroid gland, causing it to produce too much thyroid hormone.
- **Toxic Nodular Goiter**: This occurs when one or more nodules (lumps) in the thyroid gland become overactive and produce excess thyroid hormone.
- **Thyroiditis:** This is an inflammation of the thyroid gland. Certain types of thyroiditis, such as subacute thyroiditis and postpartum thyroiditis, can initially cause a temporary release of stored thyroid hormone, leading to hyperthyroidism.
- **Taking Too Much Thyroid Hormone Medication**: If you're taking medication for hypothyroidism (underactive thyroid), taking too high a dose can lead to hyperthyroidism.
- **Pituitary Tumors:** In rare cases, a noncancerous tumor in the pituitary gland can cause it to overproduce thyroid-stimulating hormone (TSH), which in turn stimulates the thyroid gland to produce too much thyroid hormone.
- **Certain Medications:** Some medications, such as amiodarone

(used to treat heart rhythm problems) and interferon-alpha (used to treat certain cancers and viral infections), can rarely cause hyperthyroidism as a side effect.

- **Excessive Iodine Intake:** While rare, consuming very high amounts of iodine can sometimes trigger hyperthyroidism in susceptible individuals.

It's important to note that the specific cause of hyperthyroidism can vary depending on the individual. If you're experiencing symptoms of hyperthyroidism, it's important to see a doctor to get a diagnosis and treatment.

DIET AND HYPERTHYROIDISM: A DEEPER DIVE

While diet itself doesn't directly cause hyperthyroidism, it can play a role in managing symptoms and potentially influencing thyroid hormone levels in certain individuals.

IODINE INTAKE

- **Importance**: Iodine is crucial for thyroid hormone production. However, excessive iodine can worsen hyperthyroidism in some cases.
- **Foods High in Iodine:**
    - **Seaweed and Kelp**: Extremely high in iodine.
    - **Iodized Salt:** A common source of excess iodine.

- **Seafood**: Cod, tuna, shrimp, and other seafood can contain significant amounts of iodine.
- **Dairy Products:** Milk and cheese can contribute to iodine intake.

- **Dietary Recommendations:**
  - If your doctor recommends it, you might need to limit your intake of iodine-rich foods.
  - Use non-iodized salt as an alternative.
  - Choose low-iodine seafood options or limit your intake of high-iodine seafood.

NUTRIENT-RICH DIET

- **Focus on Whole Foods:** A balanced diet rich in fruits, vegetables, whole grains, lean proteins, and healthy fats is essential for overall health and can support thyroid function.
- **Important Nutrients:**
  - **Selenium**: This mineral plays a crucial role in thyroid hormone metabolism. Good sources include seafood, Brazil nuts, and eggs.
  - **Zinc**: Zinc deficiency can sometimes contribute to thyroid dysfunction. Include zinc-rich foods like oysters, beef, and

pumpkin seeds in your diet.

- **Vitamin D**: Some studies suggest a link between vitamin D deficiency and thyroid disorders. Include foods like fatty fish, fortified dairy products, and egg yolks in your diet.

OTHER DIETARY CONSIDERATIONS

- **Caffeine**: Caffeine can increase heart rate and may worsen anxiety, which are common symptoms of hyperthyroidism. Limit your caffeine intake.
- **Soy**: Some studies have suggested that soy products might interfere with thyroid hormone production in some individuals. However, more research is needed.
- **Gluten**: In some cases, individuals with hyperthyroidism may also have celiac disease or non-celiac gluten sensitivity. If you suspect gluten intolerance, consult a doctor.

TREATMENT FOR HYPERTHYROIDISM

The treatment of hyperthyroidism is more complex compared to that of hypothyroidism. Treatment options include medications to inhibit thyroid function, radioactive iodine, and surgical interventions, depending on the disease's characteristics and the patient's age. However, some individuals face the possibility of a return of the condition if the medication is discontinued.

Fortunately, several effective treatment options are available. Here's a more detailed look:

ANTITHYROID MEDICATIONS

- **How they work:** These medications, such as methimazole and propylthiouracil (PTU), interfere with your thyroid gland's ability to produce hormones. Antithyroid drugs (carbimazole, propylthiouracil) are commonly indicated as a first episode in patients younger than 40 years and in those who are breastfeeding (propylthiouracil is suitable). Hypersensitivity rash (2%), agranulocytosis (0.2%), and relapse (greater than 50%) are possible disadvantages and complications of these drugs
- **Benefits:** Often the first-line treatment, especially for younger patients. They can effectively control hormone levels within a few months.
- **Considerations:**
  - May require long-term use (1-2 years or more).
  - Can have side effects like liver problems, skin rashes, and decreased white blood cell count.
  - Regular blood tests are necessary to monitor hormone levels and adjust medication dosage.

RADIOACTIVE IODINE THERAPY (RAI)

- **How it works:** You receive a single dose of radioactive iodine, which is absorbed by your thyroid gland. The radiation destroys some of the thyroid tissue.
- **Benefits:** Highly effective, often leading to a permanent cure.
- **Considerations**:
    - Can take several months for hormone levels to normalize.
    - Requires lifelong thyroid hormone replacement therapy (levothyroxine) after treatment.
    - Pregnancy and breastfeeding are contraindicated during and after treatment.

SURGERY (THYROIDECTOMY)

- **How it works:** All or part of the thyroid gland is surgically removed.
- **Benefits:** Can be a good option for large goiters, recurrent hyperthyroidism, or those with certain medical conditions.
- **Considerations:**
    - Carries surgical risks like bleeding, nerve damage, and potential for complications.
    - Requires lifelong thyroid hormone replacement therapy.

CHOOSING THE RIGHT TREATMENT

The best treatment for you depends on several factors, including:

- **Severity of hyperthyroidism:** Mild cases may be treated with medication, while more severe cases may require RAI or surgery.
- **Age and overall health:**
- **Pregnancy status:** RAI and surgery are generally avoided during pregnancy.
- **Personal preferences:** Discuss the risks and benefits of each option with your doctor to make an informed decision.

Important Considerations

- **Regular monitoring:** Regardless of the treatment chosen, regular blood tests are crucial to monitor thyroid hormone levels and adjust medication or treatment as needed.

- **Managing symptoms:** Beta-blockers can help manage rapid heart rate, anxiety, and tremors while waiting for other treatments to take effect.

- **Lifestyle factors:** A balanced diet and regular exercise can support overall health and well-being.

AYURVEDIC TREATMENT FOR HYPERTHYROIDISM

Ayurvedic management for hyperthyroidism focuses on eliminating the root cause rather than merely alleviating the symptoms. This principle aids in preventing relapse and has been shown to be more effective in hyperthyroidism when compared to modern radiotherapy, iodine supplementation, and surgical interventions; it can also be treated at the outpatient level.

It includes treatment at the *Agni* level, and medicines that possess *Pitta-Vata Shamaka* qualities are considered ideal for controlling hyperthyroidism. The dietary guidelines and proper lifestyle practices (*Dincharya* and *Ritucharya*) outlined in Ayurvedic literature should also be adhered for effective management of hyperthyroidism. **Ayurveda** suggests three essential approaches for managing any illness, namely *Nidana Parivarjana, Samsodhana Chikitsa*, and *Samshaman Chikitsa*.

NIDANA PARIVARJANA

The avoidance of various factors that cause the disease is referred to as *Nidana Parivarjana*. Hyperthyroidism arises due to *Pitta Vata vriddhi* and *Tikshnagni*. Consequently, all foods that aggravate the *Pitta Vata Dosha* should be eliminated in cases of hyperthyroidism.

SAMSHAMANA CHIKITSA (PACIFYING THERAPIES)

- *Mahatikta ghrit* and *Ksheerabala* can be consumed internally.
- Meditation, *Pranayama*, and *Yoga Asanas* play a crucial role in maintaining thyroid health.
- Yoga therapy for the gland is beneficial. Chanting '*OM*' during

meditation helps balance thyroid function. *Sheetali*, *Sheetkari*, *Nadi Shodhan*, *Bhramari*, and *Ujjayi Pranayam*, along with asanas like *Surya Namaskar* performed slowly and *Sarvangasan* can be practiced.

Some recommended foods and medicines for *Atyagni/Bhasmak Rog* include *Payasa* (milk pudding), *Krishara* (thick gruel made of rice and lentils), *Snigdha* (unctuous) products, the meat from aquatic animals or those from marshy areas and still water, and roasted sheep meat may be offered to pacify the *atyagni*.

- Thick gruel combined with ghee should be administered whenever a patient experiences hunger.
- Medicated milk combined with the *jeevaniya* group of herbs, sugar, and *ghee* may be given.
- Patients should consume *ghee* along with cold water.
- Patients might be encouraged to consume meat broth from animals living in marshy regions.

PREVENTION OF HYPERTHYROIDISM

Typically, symptoms of hyperthyroidism arise from an unhealthy diet and way of living. Consequently, hyperthyroidism can be managed to some degree by making certain adjustments in your diet and lifestyle.

- Follow a low-fat diet for thyroid-related issues.

- Incorporate more fruits and vegetables into your meals. In particular, consuming green leafy vegetables is advantageous for thyroid patients.
- Foods rich in vitamins and minerals support thyroid regulation.
- Eat more nuts such as almonds, cashews, and sunflower seeds; they provide ample copper, which is helpful for thyroid.
- Increase intake of milk and yogurt.
- Incorporate more Vitamin A into your diet.
- Avoid all junk food and foods high in preservatives.
- Practice pranayama and meditation consistently. Engage in yoga asanas.
- Strive to maintain a stress-free lifestyle & refrain from smoking, alcohol, etc.
- Eat whole grains, which are abundant in fiber, protein, and vitamins.
- The components found in licorice help maintain thyroid balance. It also hinders cancer growth in the thyroid.

NATURAL REMEDIES FOR HYPERTHYROIDISM

This condition primarily occurs due to an inadequate diet and a stressful lifestyle, leading to an imbalance of *Vata, Pitta*, and *Kapha*. In this context, Ayurvedic treatment is used to restore balance to these *Doshas*.

- Ayurvedic medicine is preferable due to its natural composition. The herbal remedies included, like *Guggulu*, *Amla*, *Kanchanar*, *Gokshura*, and *Shilajit*, are beneficial for thyroid-related ailments.
- Turmeric milk has been utilized for treating numerous health issues for ages. Likewise, consuming turmeric prepared in milk daily alleviates hyperthyroidism symptoms.
- Moreover, bottle gourd helps soothe the stomach and enhances digestive capacity. Regularly consuming bottle gourd juice also aids in mitigating hyperthyroidism.
- Combining half a spoon of aloe vera juice with two scoops of basil juice and ingesting it offers advantages, as does drinking black pepper tea.
- Taking one spoon of *Ashwagandha* powder with warm cow's milk at bedtime provides quick relief.
- The principal element, triterpenoid glyceric acid, present in licorice, is highly effective and prevents the proliferation of thyroid cancer cells.

-$$$-

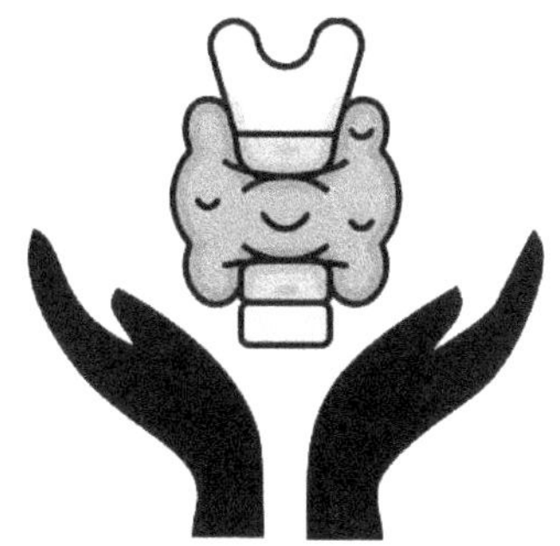

Gestational Hypothyroidism

Dr. Jyoti Kaushik, Dr Bharti Vats

Gestational Hypothyroidism (GHT) is defined as an emerging condition where insufficiency of the thyroid gland has developed during pregnancy in a previously euthyroid woman. It may be subclinical (elevated TSH and normal FT_4) or overt (Elevated TSH and low FT_4). During the few months of pregnancy, the baby relies on the mother for thyroid hormones. These hormones are vital for normal brain development and growth of the baby. Hypothyroidism in the mother can have long lasting effects on the baby.

ETIOLOGY

Gestational Hypothyroidism occur in about 2.5% of Pregnancies. The prevalence of Hypothyroidism in India is 13.13%, when ULRR (upper limit of the reference range) of TSH is set at 4.5 mIU/L, however this percentage increase upto 36.07% when ULRR is set at trimester specific reference range as suggested by ATA (American **Thyroid** Association). Endemic Iodine deficiency is the most common cause of Hypothyroidism seen in pregnant women worldwide. The clinical association of hypothyroidism in pregnancy may be due to

- First time diagnosis in pregnancy
- Hypothyroid women who either discontinue thyroid therapy or who need larger doses in pregnancy
- Hyperthyroid women on excessive amount of antithyroid drugs
- Women with lithium or amiodarone therapy.
- In Iodine sufficient environment like Hashimoto's thyroiditis, surgical ablation of Grave's disease, Prior radioactive Iodine treatment, thyroidectomy, Sheehan's Syndrome.
- Medications like Thionamides, Lithium, Ferrous sulphate, Cholestyramine, Antacids like Aluminium hydroxide.

Table: Normal Range of Thyroid Levels In Pregnancy

Normal Range	First Trimester	Second Trimester	Third Trimester
T3 (ng/mL)	1.21 to 1.32	1.13 to 1.64	1.16 to 1.51
T4 (µg/dL)	7.57 to 8.13	7.17 to 8.64	7.07 to 8.44
TSH (uIU/mL)	0.18 to 2.99	0.11 to 3.98	0.48 to 4.71

According to the guidelines of American Thyroid Association in 2017, the upper limit of reference range of TSH during First Trimester to be set at 4 mIU/L and for 2nd and 3rd trimester is same as general population.

EFFECT OF PREGNANCY ON THYROID PHYSIOLOGY

During pregnancy, thyroid hormone production increases by around 50% along with a similar increase in total daily iodine requirements. Iodine is an essential component of the thyroid hormones, triiodothyronine (T3) and thyroxine (T4), produced by the thyroid gland. The fetal thyroid does not begin to concentrate iodine until 10–12 weeks of gestation, and the synthesis and secretion of thyroid hormone controlled by fetal pituitary thyroid stimulating hormone (TSH) ensues at approximately 20 weeks of gestation. As such, particularly during early pregnancy, the fetus is reliant on maternal thyroxine, which cross the placenta in small quantities to maintain normal fetal thyroid function. At birth, approximately 30% of the T4 in cord blood originates from the infant's mother.

During Pregnancy, maternal thyroid function is modulated by three factors:

- An increase in HCG concentration that stimulate the thyroid gland.
- Significant increases in urinary iodide excretion resulting in a fall

in Plasma lodide Concentration.

- An increase in thyroxine – binding globulin(TBG) during the first trimester, resulting in increased binding of thyroxine.

EFFECT OF HCG ON THYROID

Thyroid function tests change during normal pregnancy due to the influence of two main hormones:

- Human chorionic gonadotropin (hCG)
- Estrogen.

TSH is a glycoprotein consisting of two subunits alfa and beta. Alfa subunits is identical to hCG and beta subunit is unique to TSH. So, hCG mimics and acts like TSH. It binds to the TSH receptor on the thyroid cell membrane and is a weak stimulator, resulting in increased secretion of T4 and T3 and partial suppression of serum TSH. The high circulating hCG levels in the first trimester may result in a low TSH and may even be below the lower limit of 0.4 mIU/L. Since the level of hCG decrease as the pregnancy increases, the level of TSH follows the reverse trend. The higher serum hCG concentrations seen in multiple gestation pregnancies is associated with an even greater degree of TSH suppression; maternal serum TSH concentrations are lower in twin pregnancies, compared to a singleton pregnancy, and even lower in triplet or quadruplet pregnancies

Estrogen increases the amount of thyroid hormone binding

proteins, and this increases the total thyroid hormone levels but the "Free" hormone (the amount that is not bound and can be active for use) usually remains normal. The thyroid is functioning normally if the TSH and Free T4 remain in the trimester-specific normal ranges throughout pregnancy.

EFFECT OF INCREASED URINARY IODIDE EXCRETION

Enhanced metabolism of T_4 in the second and third trimester, due to a rise in placental type 2 and type 3 deiodinases which convert T_4 to T_3 and T_4 to reverse T_3 and T_2 respectively, act as further impact to T_4 synthesis. Plasma iodide levels decrease due to both increased thyroxine metabolism and increased renal iodide clearance.

All these changes lead to increase in the size of the thyroid gland in 15% of Pregnant women, which return to normal in the Post Partum Period.

EFFECT OF INCREASED THYROXINE BINDING GLOBULIN(TBG)

T3 is the active thyroid hormone, and approximately 80% of T3 is produced from the deiodination of T4 in the liver, muscle, and other tissues. The binding of T3 to thyroid hormone receptors in various peripheral target tissues are important for the regulation of the body's metabolism. Approximately 99.97% of T4 and 99.7% of T3 is protein-bound, primarily to thyroid hormone binding globulin (TBG), and in lesser amounts, to albumin and transthyretin (the latter for T4 only).

Beginning in early pregnancy, rising maternal estradiol levels result in increased sialyation and glycosylation of TBG in the liver. This decreases the peripheral metabolism of TBG to result in an approximate 1.5–2 fold sustained rise in serum TBG levels compared to euthyroid non-pregnant women, thereby creating an increased need for T3 and T4 production throughout pregnancy.

PHYSIOLOGICAL CHANGES IN THYROID HORMONE DURING PREGNANCY

Pregnancy significantly impacts thyroid hormone levels and function in a woman's body. Here's a breakdown of the key changes:

1. INCREASED THYROID HORMONE DEMAND:

- **Fetal Development:** The fetus relies on the mother's thyroid hormones for early brain development.
- **Placental Needs:** The placenta also requires thyroid hormones for its proper function.

2. HORMONAL INFLUENCES:

- **Human Chorionic Gonadotropin (hCG):** This pregnancy hormone, produced by the placenta, has a similar structure to thyroid-stimulating hormone (TSH). In early pregnancy, hCG can mildly stimulate the thyroid gland, leading to a slight increase in thyroid hormone production.
- **Estrogen:** Estrogen levels rise significantly during pregnancy.

This increases the production of thyroxine-binding globulin (TBG), a protein that binds to thyroid hormones in the blood.

3. CHANGES IN THYROID HORMONE LEVELS:

- **Total T4 and T3:** Due to the increase in TBG, the total levels of T4 (thyroxine) and T3 (triiodothyronine) in the blood typically rise during pregnancy.
- **Free T4 and T3:** While total levels increase, the levels of *free* T4 and T3 (the biologically active forms of the hormones) may remain relatively stable or slightly decrease.

4. TSH LEVELS:

- **Early Pregnancy:** TSH levels may slightly decrease due to the effects of hCG.
- **Later Pregnancy:** TSH levels generally increase as pregnancy progresses.

IODINE REQUIREMENT IN PREGNANCY

Iodine is an element essential for normal growth and for the development of the brain. Iodine deficiency is the most common cause of thyroid disease, specifically hypothyroidism (underactive thyroid). Iodine deficiency is usually treated by eating more iodine-rich salt, using iodised salt and taking iodine supplements.

Table: Physiological Changes In Thyroid Hormone

Maternal Status	Pregnancy	Hyperthyroidism	Hypothyroidism
TSH	No change	Decrease	Increase
Free T4	No change	Increase	Decrease
Free Thyroxine Index (FTI)	No change	Increase	Decrease
Total T4	Increase	Increase	Decrease
Total T3	Increase	Increase or No change	Decrease or No change
Resin Triiodo-thyronine Uptake (RT3U)	Decrease	Increase	Decrease

DAILY REQUIREMENT OF IODINE

- for women planning Pregnancy – 150 µg/day
- for Pregnant women – 220 µg/day
- for Lactating Mother – 290 µg/day

Iodine required for infant's nutrition, is secreted into breast milk. Therefore, lactating women also have increased dietary iodine requirements. The World Health Organization (WHO) and American Thyroid Agency (ATA) recommends that all Pregnant and Lactating women ingest a minimum of 250 µg/day Iodine optimally in the form of Potassium Iodide during Pregnancy and Lactation.

CLASSIFICATION OF GESTATIONAL HYPOTHYROIDISM

1.OVERT HYPOTHYROIDISM

It is defined as raised TSH above the upper limit of normal and a free T_4 below the lower limit of normal. The consensus from professional societies including ATA, endocrine society and the American Association of Clinical Endocrinologist (AACE) is that any women with TSH > 10 mIU even with normal free T_4 should be diagnosed as Overt Hypothyroidism.

2.SUBCLINICAL HYPOTHYROIDISM

Subclinical hypothyroidism is defined as a high TSH and normal T4 concentration. Its prevalence in pregnancy has been estimated to be 2-5%. It is more common in women particularly those who have thyroid antibodies. It is unlikely to progress to hypothyroidism during pregnancy in otherwise healthy women but is increasingly being discussed as adverse maternal and fetal outcomes have been observed. In a study it is found that, its progression to hypothyroidism occurred more often in patients whose ultrasonographic thyroid scan showed diffuse hypo-echogenicity (an indication of chronic thyroiditis).

A Randomized Trial of Thyroxine Therapy for Subclinical Hypothyroidism or hypothyroxinaemia diagnosed during pregnancy demonstrated no difference in neurocognitive development in offspring through age 5 years who were born to women screened and treated for Subclinical hypothyroidism. Moreover, follow-up of children through age 9 years confirmed that there was no neurodevelopmental improvement in offspring of treated women.

Diagnosis is essentially a biochemical one as symptoms may be mild, nonspecific, or even absent. In pregnancy, its diagnosis is often incidental. Higher TSH and higher SCH prevalence level are consistently seen in those who are TPO-Ab or TgAb positive.

3.ISOLATED HYPOTHYROXINAEMIA

It is typically defined as a FT_4 concentration in the lower 2.5^{th} to 5th percentile of a given population in conjunction with a normal maternal TSH concentration.

SYMPTOMS OF GESTATIONAL HYPOTHYROIDISM

Gestational hypothyroidism can sometimes be difficult to recognize because many of its symptoms overlap with common pregnancy discomforts. Here are some of the potential symptoms:

- **Fatigue:** Feeling unusually tired or lacking energy is a common symptom of both pregnancy and hypothyroidism.
- **Weight gain:** While some weight gain is expected during pregnancy, excessive weight gain or difficulty losing weight may be a sign of hypothyroidism.
- **Constipation:** Hormonal changes during pregnancy can cause

constipation, but it can also be a symptom of hypothyroidism.

- **Intolerance to cold:** Feeling unusually cold, even in warm temperatures, can be a sign of an underactive thyroid.
- **Depression:** While pregnancy can bring on emotional changes, persistent feelings of sadness, anxiety, or hopelessness may be a sign of hypothyroidism.
- **Muscle aches and weakness:** Hypothyroidism can cause muscle weakness and stiffness.
- **Hair loss:** Thinning hair or hair loss is a common symptom of hypothyroidism.
- **Dry skin:** Hypothyroidism can cause dry, flaky skin.
- **Hoarse voice:** Changes in voice quality can sometimes occur with hypothyroidism.
- **Menstrual irregularities:** While menstrual cycles typically stop during pregnancy, irregular periods before conception can be a sign of an underlying thyroid issue.

SCREENING FOR THYROID DISORDERS

Routine screening has been recommended as per American thyroid association 2017 guidelines-

- In case of Infertility, Menstrual Disorders, Repeated Pregnancy loss, Type 1 Diabetes Mellitus

- Pregnant women who have signs and symptoms of deficient thyroid function.
- A women having history of Hypothyroidism/Hyperthyroidism.
- Known thyroid antibody positivity or presence of a goiter.
- History of head or neck radiation or prior thyroid surgery.
- A women having age > 30 years
- A women having multiple prior pregnancies, more than 2.
- Family history of Autoimmune thyroid disease or thyroid disfunction.
- Morbid obesity (BMI body mass index 40kg/m^2)
- Use of Amiodarone or Lithium, or recent administration of iodinated radiologic contrast.
- Residing in an area of known moderate to severe iodine insufficiency.

LABORATORY TESTS

Because screening is controversial and symptomatology does not reliably distinguish hypothyroidism from normal pregnancy, laboratory tests are the standard for diagnosis.

1. **Overt Hypothyroidism**
    - Symptomatic Patient
    - Elevated TSH level
    - Low level of FT_4 and FT_3.

2. **Subclinical Hypothyroidism**
    - Asymptomatic Patient
    - Elevated TSH level
    - Normal FT_4 and FT_3.

EFFECT OF HYPOTHYROIDISM ON MOTHER

Untreated or inadequately treated hypothyroidism during pregnancy can have several negative effects on the mother:

- **Increased risk of miscarriage:** One of the most significant risks, especially in the first trimester.
- **Premature birth:** Increased likelihood of delivering the baby before 37 weeks of gestation.
- **Preeclampsia:** A serious condition characterized by high blood pressure and organ damage.
- **Placental problems:** Potentially leading to complications like placental abruption (where the placenta separates from the uterine wall).
- **Postpartum hemorrhage:** Increased risk of excessive bleeding after delivery.
- **Gestational diabetes:** A higher chance of developing gestational diabetes occurs during pregnancy.
- **Heart problems:** In severe cases, potential for heart-related complications.

EFFECT OF HYPOTHYROIDISM ON FETUS

Fetus requires maternal thyroxin/T_4 for normal brain development before 12 weeks. Inadequate replacement may lead to reduced neuro-psychological development of the offspring. It is rare for maternal thyroid inhibitory antibodies to cross the placenta and cause fetal Hypothyroidism.

Untreated or inadequately treated hypothyroidism during pregnancy can have significant and potentially irreversible effects on the developing fetus, primarily impacting brain development. Here's a more detailed look:

1. IMPAIRED BRAIN DEVELOPMENT

- **Crucial Role of Thyroid Hormones:** Thyroid hormones are absolutely vital for the proper development of the fetal brain. They play a critical role in:
- **Cell growth and differentiation:** Thyroid hormones regulate the growth and specialization of brain cells.
    - **Myelination:** This process involves the formation of a protective sheath around nerve fibers, crucial for efficient nerve signal transmission.
    - **Synapse formation:** The connections between brain cells are essential for proper brain function.

- **Cognitive Impairment:** Children born to mothers with untreated hypothyroidism may experience:
    - Lower IQ
    - Learning difficulties
    - Delayed speech and language development
    - Attention and behavioral problems
- **Motor Impairment:**
    - Delayed motor skills, such as crawling, walking, and fine motor skills.
- **Neurological Issues:**
    - Potential for more severe neurological problems in severe cases.

2. OTHER POTENTIAL EFFECTS

- **Growth Restriction:** The fetus may experience slowed growth, resulting in low birth weight.
- **Premature Birth:** Increased risk of delivering the baby before 37 weeks of gestation.
- **Increased Risk of Other Complications:** Although less common, potential for other developmental problems.

MANAGEMENT OF GESTATIONAL HYPOTHYROIDISM

PRE-PREGNANCY COUNSELLING

- Counselling of the patients with known hypothyroidism should be done to optimize medical therapy and delay pregnancy until TSH level of <2.5 mIU/L is achieved before pregnancy.
- Dose of levothyroxine is adjusted so as to to achieve a value between the lower reference range limit and 2.5 mIU/L.
- Patient receiving Levothyroxine, with a suspected pregnancy should independently adjust their dose of Levothyroxine, by 20-30% and immediately notify their doctor for further evaluation. One means of accomplishing this is to take two additional tablets weekly of the patient's current daily Levothyroxine dose.
- Counsel the patient regarding increased demand of thyroxine during pregnancy.

MANAGEMENT DURING PREGNANCY

Overt maternal hypothyroidism should be treated and diagnosed as early as possible because it is known to have serious effects on the fetus.

- The drug of choice is levothyroxine and the dose should be adjusted so as to keep the serum TSH below 2.5 mIU/L in the first trimester or 3 mIU/L in second and third trimesters. The aim is to maintain Free Thyroxine, at the upper end of the normal range and TSH in the trimester-specific normal range.

- Many clinical studies have proved that the increased requirement of thyroxine occurs as early as 4-6 weeks of pregnancy and it gradually increases through 16-20 weeks of pregnancy and plateau thereafter until delivery.
- In pregnant women with previously diagnosed hypothyroidism, serum TSH levels should be measured every 3-4 weeks during the first half of pregnancy and every 6-10 weeks thereafter. After every dosage adjustment, TSH and free Thyroxine levels should be measured after 3-4 weeks.

AUTOIMMUNE THYROID DISEASE

- Autoimmune thyroid disease has been associated with a higher miscarriage rate.
- Anti-TPO or anti-Tg thyroid autoantibodies are present in 2-17% of unselected pregnant women.
- A study from Belgium in women taking fertility treatment showed that both TPO-Ab and thyroglobulin antibody (TgAb) were present in 8% of women, while 5% showed isolated TgAbs and 4% showed isolated TPO-Ab concentrations. The women with isolated Tg-Ab had a significantly higher serum TSH than women without thyroid autoimmunity.
- A study showed that women with anti-TPO antibodies who were

treated with Levothyroxine, during the first trimester had lower miscarriage and premature delivery rates than those who were not treated.

DOSE OF LEVOTHYROXINE

- To return the patients to a euthyroid state, the most successful dosages, as follow, varied according to baseline levels of TSH:
    - Subclinical Hypothyroidism (TSH 4.2 mIU/L or less): 1.2 µg/kg/day
    - Subclinical Hypothyroidism (TSH>4.2-10 mIU/L): 1.42 µg/kg/day
    - Overt Hypothyroidism: 2.33 µg/kg/day
- According to ACOG (American College of Obstetricians and Gynaecologists) recommendation: Initial dose 1-2 µg/kg daily or 100 µg. Further adjustment is made according to TSH level as follows:
    - If TSH level is elevated but <10 mIU/L, add 25-50 µg/day
    - If TSH level is >10 mIU/L, but <20 mIU/L, add 50-75 µg/day
    - If TSH level is >20 mIU/L, then add 75-100 µg/day.

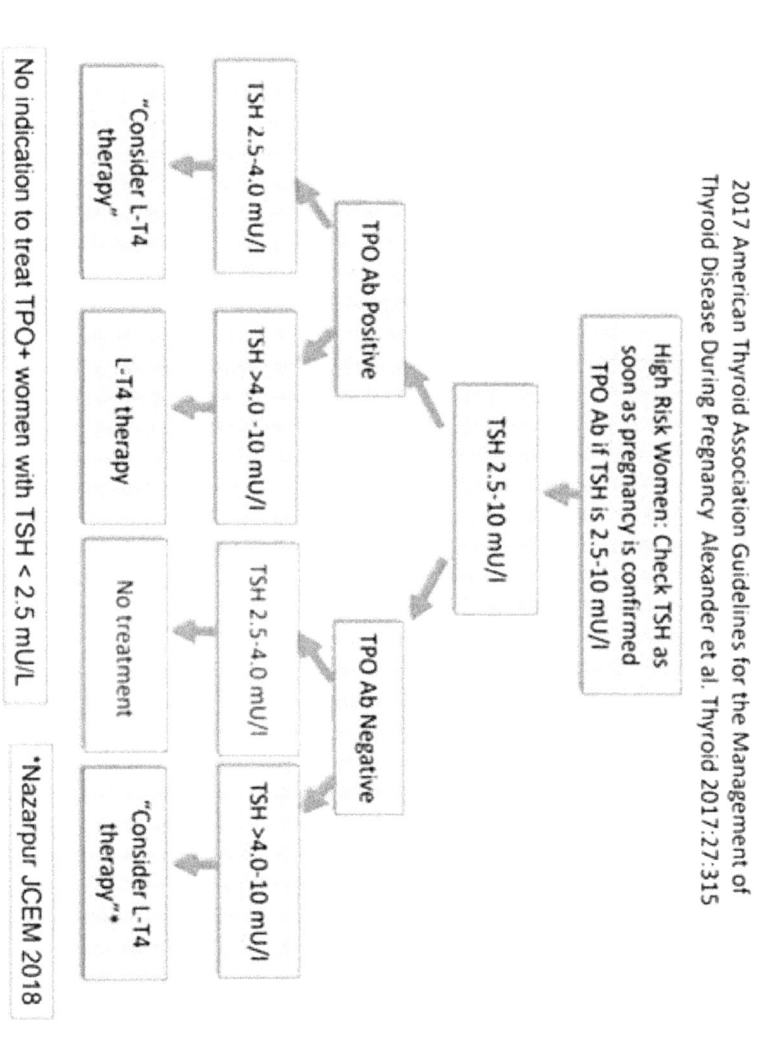
2017 American Thyroid Association Guidelines for the Management of Thyroid Disease During Pregnancy Alexander et al. Thyroid 2017:27:315
High Risk Women: Check TSH as soon as pregnancy is confirmed TPO Ab if TSH is 2.5-10 mU/l
TSH 2.5-10 mU/l
TPO Ab Positive
TPO Ab Negative
TSH 2.5-4.0 mU/l
TSH >4.0 -10 mU/l
TSH 2.5-4.0 mU/l
TSH >4.0-10 mU/l
"Consider L-T4 therapy"
L-T4 therapy
No treatment
"Consider L-T4 therapy"*
No indication to treat TPO+ women with TSH < 2.5 mU/L
*Nazarpur JCEM 2018

- After adjustment of the dose, TSH should be checked in every trimester to maintain euthyroid. Women having thyroid autoimmunity who are euthyroid in the early stages of pregnancy are at risk of developing hypothyroidism and should be monitored every 4-6 weeks for elevation of TSH above the normal range for pregnancy.
- Levothyroxine should not be taken with iron, vitamins, or calcium supplements as these may reduce its absorption.

MANAGEMENT DURING LABOR AND DELIVERY

- In a well-controlled patient, no specific measures are necessary. Large maternal goitre may cause anaesthetic complications in case of general anaesthesia (GA) if needed.

POSTNATAL MANAGEMENT

- After delivery, the dose should be reduced to pre pregnancy regimen. TSH should be checked at 6 weeks postpartum.
- Signs of postpartum thyroiditis should be checked and the patient should be screened for postpartum depression.

SCREENING AND MANAGEMENT OF CONGENITAL HYPOTHYROIDISM IN NEONATES:

- Two to five days after birth, all newborns should be screened for congenital hypothyroidism by using cord blood, or postnatal blood ideally at 48-72 hours of age in order to avoid confounding by the physiologic surge in neonatal TSH.

- Neonates with screen TSFI >20 mIU/L or >34 mIU/L for samples taken between 24 and 48 hours of age should be recalled for confirmation by venous blood.

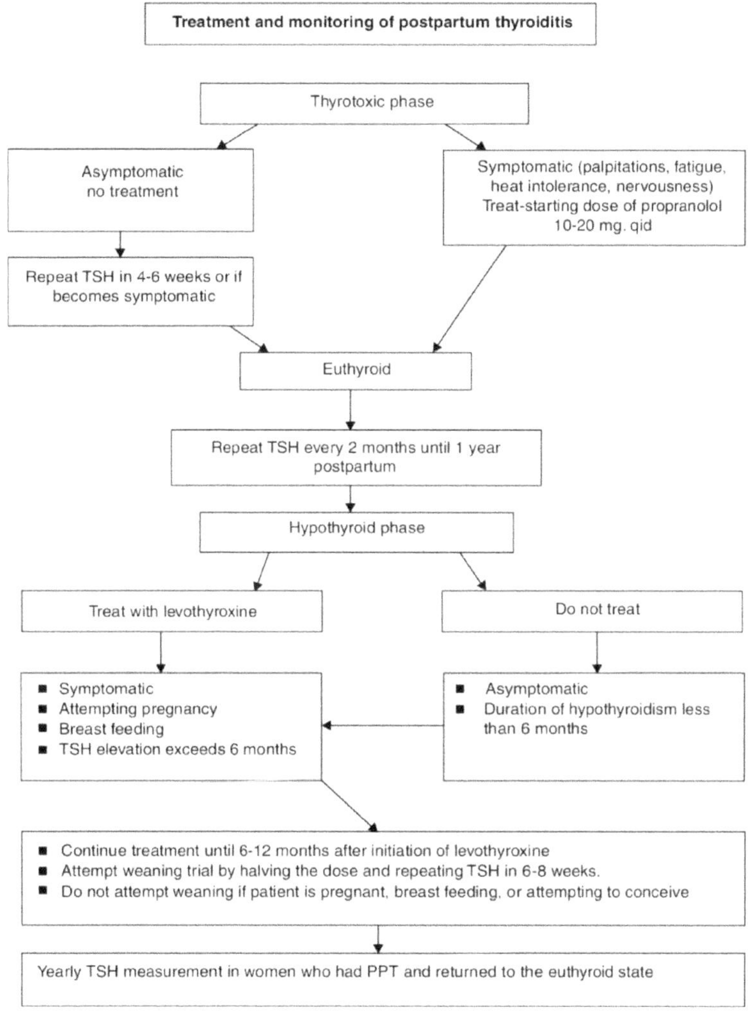

- Venous confirmatory TSH >20 mIU/L before age 2 weeks and >10 mIU/L age 2 weeks, with low T4 (< 10 ug/dl) or FT 4 (< 1.17ng /dL) indicate primary congenital hypothyroidism.
- **Treatment** - Neonates with congenital hypothyroidism, Levothyroxine should be started within 2 weeks of life at a dose of 10 – 15 ug /day for a term baby. In case of a premature baby, lower dose should be taken.
- Serum T4 should be measured at 2 weeks and TSH and T4 at 1 month, then 2 monthly till 6 months, 3 monthly from 6 months to 3 years and every 3-6 months thereafter. Babies with the possibility of transient congenital hypothyroidism should be re-evaluated at age 3 years, to assess the need for lifelong therapy.

AYURVEDIC MANAGEMENT

- **Herbal Remedies:** Ayurvedic herbs like Ashwagandha, Guggulu, Brahmi and Mandukaparni possess adaptogenic and hormone-balancing properties, helping regulate thyroid hormone production and support overall thyroid function.
- **Dietary Modifications:** Ayurveda recommends a thyroid-supportive diet that includes iodine-rich foods like yogurt, and fresh vegetables. It also suggests minimizing processed foods, refined sugars, and stimulants like caffeine, which can negatively impact thyroid function.

- **Stress Management:** Ayurveda recognizes the link between stress and thyroid health. Stress-reducing practices such as meditation, yoga, pranayama, breathing exercises, are recommended to support overall well-being and promote hormonal balance.
- **Lifestyle Adjustments:** Ayurveda suggests maintaining a regular daily routine, getting adequate sleep, and engaging in gentle exercise to enhance energy flow, support digestion, and promote hormonal equilibrium.

-$$$-

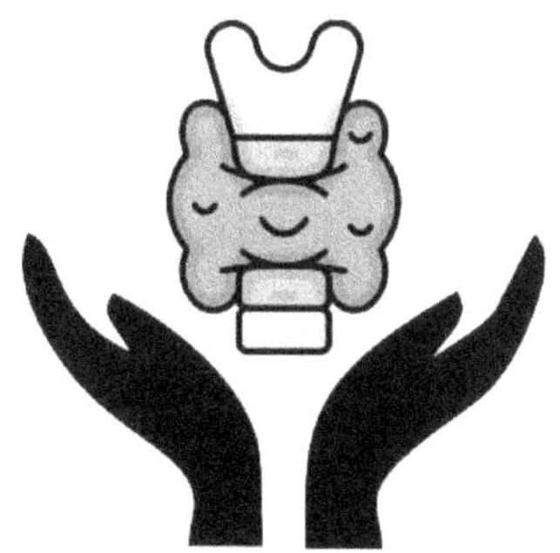

Balancing Your Thyroid

Dr. Tina Singhal

Thyroid problems, such as hypothyroidism and hyperthyroidism, are becoming more common in today's fast-moving society. While contemporary medicine treats these disorders with hormone therapy and other methods, **Ayurveda** adopts a holistic viewpoint by prioritizing the balance of the body's energies, referred to as '*Doshas*', and fostering prolonged health. This time-honoured healing practice, rooted in ancient texts such as the **Charak Samhita** and **Sushrut Samhita**, perceives the thyroid gland as indicative of the body's overall equilibrium and metabolic wellness.

While they don't explicitly mention Ayurvedic treatment for *overt* hypothyroidism, they extensively discuss the efficacy of various Ayurvedic herbs in managing subclinical hypothyroidism (SCH). In **Ayurveda**, the functionality of the thyroid gland is intricately linked to the throat *chakra (Vishuddha)* and the interactions between the *Kapha* and *Pitta Doshas*. When these *Doshas* experience imbalance, it may result in an underactive thyroid (hypothyroidism) or an overactive thyroid (hyperthyroidism). The Ayurvedic methodology not only seeks to re-establish hormonal balance but also considers factors such as lifestyle, dietary habits, and mental health. It is important to note that the following discussion focuses primarily on the Ayurvedic management of SCH.

SUBCLINICAL HYPOTHYROIDISM (SCH)

SCH represents a milder form of hypothyroidism where serum TSH levels are elevated, but free T_3 (FT_3) and free T_4 (FT_4) levels remain within the normal range. This indicates early thyroid failure, but individuals may experience mild symptoms or remain asymptomatic.

THE AYURVEDIC PERSPECTIVE

Ayurveda views hypothyroidism through the lens of *Agnimandya*, which signifies low metabolic activity at both the systemic and cellular levels. This can be understood as a state of reduced caloric expenditure or hypometabolism in modern terms. According to **Ayurveda**, *Agnimandya* is often triggered by factors that increase *Kapha Dosha*, leading to an accumulation of metabolic waste products at the cellular level (*Dhatugata Mala Sanchaya*). This build-up obstructs microchannels (*Srotorodha*), hindering the flow of nutrients and energy, ultimately affecting the essence of body tissues.

Hypothyroidism manifests when the thyroid gland slows down, usually due to a *Kapha Dosha* imbalance. This leads to symptoms such as fatigue, weight gain, constipation, and depression. **Ayurveda** interprets this situation as a buildup of heaviness and coldness within the body, necessitating treatments that invigorate the digestive fire (*Agni*) and eliminate blockages.

Conversely, hyperthyroidism, linked with *Pitta* imbalance, precipitates excessive metabolic activity. Symptoms encompass anxiety, significant weight loss, intolerance to heat, and palpitations. **Ayurveda** acknowledges this as an overstimulation of heat and energy, requiring cooling and soothing interventions.

AYURVEDIC TREATMENT STRATEGIES FOR SCH

Various studies highlight a wide array of Ayurvedic herbs and formulations that have shown potential in managing SCH. The treatment strategies generally aim to:

- **Stimulate Thyroid Hormone Production:** Some herbs are believed to directly or indirectly enhance the production of thyroid hormones, thus addressing the deficiency.
- **Improve Metabolism and Energy Production:** Ayurvedic formulations often incorporate herbs that stimulate digestion and metabolism (*Deepana* and *Pachana*), thereby improving *Agni*

and counteracting *Agnimandya*.

- **Clear Microchannels:** Herbs with *Srotoshodhaka* properties are used to remove blockages in the body's microchannels, facilitating the smooth flow of nutrients and energy.
- **Reduce Excess Kapha and Fat:** Formulations often include herbs that possess *Medohara* and *Lekhana* properties to reduce excess *Kapha* and lipids, addressing weight gain associated with SCH.

COMPREHENSIVE AYURVEDIC TREATMENT

Ayurvedic therapy for thyroid disorders takes a holistic approach that goes beyond just targeting the thyroid gland itself. Instead, it centers on harmonizing the entire body, mind, and spirit. This all-encompassing approach involves tailored herbal preparations, detoxification methods like *Panchakarma*, dietary modifications, and adjustments to lifestyle.

DETOXIFICATION THROUGH PANCHAKARMA

Among the most effective techniques in **Ayurveda** for tackling thyroid disorders is Panchakarma, a sequence of detoxifying and revitalizing treatments. These therapies eliminate built-up toxins (*Ama*) that hinder the optimal functioning of the thyroid gland.

For hypothyroidism, techniques such as *Vamana* (therapeutic vomiting) and *Basti* (medicated enema) are employed to remove excess *Kapha* and stimulate metabolism. In cases of hyperthyroidism, *Virechana* (therapeutic purgation) is suggested to balance *Pitta* and diminish the surplus heat in the body. *Panchakarma* not only detoxifies but also rejuvenates the entire system, re-establishing balance to the *Doshas* and enhancing overall wellness.

LIFESTYLE ADJUSTMENTS FOR THYROID HEALTH

In **Ayurveda**, lifestyle modifications are deemed vital for healing and sustaining thyroid health. These adaptations are customized to fit each person's distinct constitution and *Dosha* imbalances. For thyroid conditions, the following essential lifestyle changes are advised:

1. Daily Routine (Dincharya): Adhering to a consistent daily pattern, or *dincharya*, aids in maintaining bodily balance. This includes rising early, engaging in oil pulling for detoxification, and maintaining a regular schedule for meals and rest.

2. Yoga and Meditation: Certain yoga poses and breathing exercises can enhance thyroid health by boosting circulation and activating the endocrine system. Asanas like *Sarvangasana* (Shoulder Stand), *Matsyasana* (Fish Pose), and *Halasana* (Plow Pose) are recognized for their direct effect on the thyroid gland. In addition, meditation aids in stress reduction, which significantly influences both hypothyroidism and hyperthyroidism.

3. Stress Management: In **Ayurveda**, stress is regarded as a key factor in causing imbalances in the body, especially relating to thyroid disorders. Techniques such as mindfulness meditation, **pranayama** (breathing exercises), and spending time outdoors can assist in alleviating stress and enhancing thyroid function.

AYURVEDIC DIET

The Ayurvedic approach to treating thyroid disorders through diet is based on balancing specific *Doshas* associated with each condition.

Hypothyroidism is linked to an imbalance in the *Kapha Dosha*. To address this, **Ayurveda** suggests consuming warming, invigorating foods that stimulate digestion and metabolism.

- **Spices** such as **ginger, cumin, and black pepper** are recommended for improving digestion and boosting metabolism.
- **Millets, barley, and quinoa**, considered light and easily digestible grains, are believed to stimulate digestive fire.
- **Leafy greens and cruciferous vegetables** are recommended for their detoxification properties and thyroid-stimulating effects, although they should be thoroughly cooked.
- **Sesame oil and ghee** are considered nourishing yet light, promoting Agni (digestive fire) stimulation without burdening the digestive system.
- **Hyperthyroidism**, on the other hand, is associated with an excess of the ***Pitta Dosha***. To balance this, **Ayurveda**

emphasizes cooling, soothing foods that reduce heat in the body.

- **Cooling foods** like cucumber, melons, and avocados are recommended to alleviate excess heat.
- **Coconut water** is valued for its cooling properties and its ability to balance ***Pitta***.
- **Bitter greens** such as dandelion greens and kale are believed to reduce ***Pitta***'s overactivity.
- **Cooling dairy products** like milk and ghee are suggested in moderation to help mitigate excess heat.

The information presented here is based solely on the various researches and does not constitute medical advice. It is essential to consult with a qualified healthcare professional for diagnosis and treatment of thyroid disorders.

A CLOSER LOOK AT HERBAL REMEDIES

This Section focus on exploring the potential of Ayurvedic herbs in managing hypothyroidism, particularly subclinical hypothyroidism (SCH). While **Ayurveda** doesn't have a specific term for thyroid gland, but a condition called *Galaganda* that shares symptomatic similarities with thyroid disorders. This review focuses on how various herbs can help manage hypothyroidism by stimulating thyroid hormone production, improving metabolism, clearing microchannels, and reducing excess *Kapha* and fat.

HERBAL REMEDIES AND THEIR PROPOSED MECHANISMS

This section discuss various herbal remedies and their potential benefits in managing SCH. Here is a closer look at some of the key herbs:

- **Brahmi (Bacopa monnieri):** Brahmi is a well-known herb in Ayurvedic medicine. Studies suggest that Brahmi leaf extract can **increase T_4 levels** in mice, possibly by **directly stimulating the thyroid gland** or **enhancing T4 conversion**. This suggests that Brahmi could potentially play a role in managing hypothyroidism by addressing the hormone deficiency.
- **Nigella sativa:** This herb, also known as Kalonji, is known for its **antioxidant properties**. The studies highlight its ability to **protect against learning and memory impairment** and **hormonal imbalances** associated with hypothyroidism in animal models.
- **Curcuma longa (Turmeric):** Curcumin, the active compound in turmeric, is widely recognized for its potent **anti-inflammatory and antioxidant effects**. Research indicates that curcumin can **improve antioxidant defenses in the brain**, potentially **counteracting the oxidative stress** induced by hypothyroidism.
- **Fruit Peel Extracts:** Extracts from the peels of mango (Mangifera indica), muskmelon (Cucumis melo), and watermelon (Citrullus

vulgaris) have shown promising results in **restoring T3 and T4 levels** in rats with hypothyroidism. This suggests they might have **thyroid-stimulating properties**. However, the various studies recommend using these extracts individually, as combined use might increase lipid peroxidation.

- **Crataeva nurvala (Varuna):** Varuna extract has demonstrated a potential role in managing hypothyroidism. Studies show it can **increase free T_4 levels** and **decrease TSH levels** in a dose-dependent manner, suggesting it might help regulate thyroid hormone production.
- **Costus pictus (Insulin Plant):** The insulin plant has garnered attention for its potential antidiabetic effects. Research suggests that its extract can also **restore thyroid hormone levels**, **reduce TSH** and have **beneficial effects on cholesterol and inflammation**.
- **Withania somnifera (Ashwagandha) and Bauhinia purpurea (Kovidara):** Both Ashwagandha and Kovidara are commonly used in Ayurvedic practices. Studies highlight their ability to **restore T3 and T4 levels** in diabetic mice experiencing hypothyroidism, suggesting a potential role in managing hypothyroidism in specific populations.
- **Bauhinia variegata (Kanchanara)** and **Eichhornia crassipes (Jalakumbhi):** Kanchanara and Jalakumbhi extracts have

exhibited thyroid-stimulating effects in animal studies. They have shown potential in improving thyroid function and reducing cholesterol levels in hypothyroid rats.

- **Commiphora mukul (Guggulu):** Guggulu, a resin widely used in Ayurvedic formulations, has shown promising results in **increasing T3 levels** and **improving food consumption** in mice. This suggests it might have a role in addressing the metabolic slowdown associated with hypothyroidism.
- **Achyranthes aspera (Apamarga):** Apamarga leaf extract has shown **thyroid-stimulating properties**, demonstrated by **increased T3 and T4 levels** in rats. The associated increase in blood glucose further supports its potential role in boosting metabolism.
- **Saussurea lappa (Kustha)** and **Inula racemosa (Pushkaramoola):** Extracts of Kustha and Pushkaramoola have exhibited **mild thyroid-stimulating effects** in rats, as observed through thyroid histology. However, some studies suggest that their efficacy might be lower compared to other herbs.
- **Moringa oleifera (Shigru):** Moringa, known for its nutritional value, has also shown potential in regulating hypothyroidism. Studies using Moringa leaf aqueous extract in rats have demonstrated **increases in T_3 and T_4 levels** and **decreases in TSH levels**, indicating a potential for thyroid hormone regulation.

- **Ficus carica (Phalgu):** Ficus carica leaf extract, commonly known as fig, has been reported to have a positive effect on thyroid hormone levels. The presence of **tyrosine**, a precursor to thyroid hormones, in fig is suggested as a possible contributing factor.

AYURVEDIC FORMULATIONS

- **Vyoshadi Guggulu and Shadushana Churna:** This study mention a pilot clinical trial that investigated these formulations' effectiveness in managing SCH. The study reported **significant reductions in serum TSH levels and BMI** with no adverse effects. However, further research with larger sample sizes is needed to confirm these findings.

-$$$-

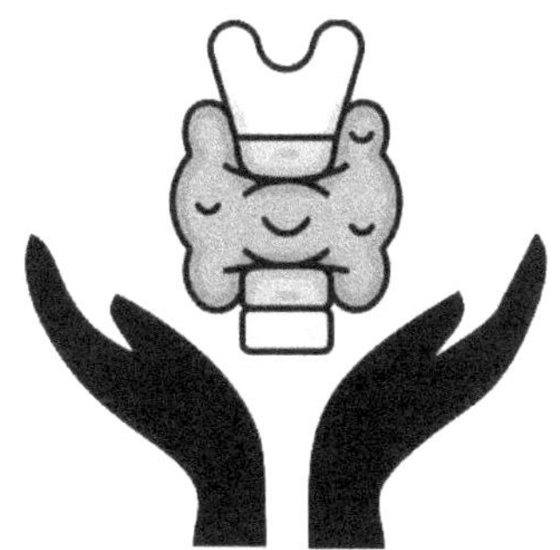

Panchakarma in Thyroid Disorder

Dr. Abhishek Yadav

Panchakarma means *five actions* or *five treatments* in Sanskrit, referring to the five major processes designed to detoxify the body. These processes aim to remove toxins (ama) from the body and harmonize the three *Doshas (Vata, Pitta,* and *Kapha),* which are thought to control bodily functions.

VAMANA (EMESIS THERAPY)

Purpose: To eliminate excess *Kapha Dosha.*

Procedure: The patient receives certain medications and herbal formulations to trigger vomiting. This aids in clearing surplus mucus and toxins from the upper gastrointestinal tract, lungs, and respiratory system. *Vamana* is generally recommended for ailments like asthma, skin problems, GI disorders and allergies.

VIRECHANA (PURGATION THERAPY)

Purpose: To eradicate excess *Pitta Dosha*.

Procedure: Laxatives or purgative herbs are provided to cleanse the small intestine and detoxify the liver and gallbladder. This technique effectively addresses skin disorders, jaundice, gastrointestinal problems, and inflammatory conditions. It assists in regulating digestion and metabolism.

BASTI (ENEMA THERAPY)

Purpose: To equilibrate ***Vata Dosha***.

Procedure: Medicated enemas are administered to purify the colon. Various types of *Basti* exist, including *Anuvasana Basti* (oil enema) and *Niruha Basti* (decoction enema). This treatment is advantageous for constipation, arthritis, neurological issues, and lower back pain. It helps to remove deeply embedded toxins and enhances gut health.

NASYA (NASAL ADMINISTRATION)

Purpose: To eliminate toxins from the head and neck area.

Procedure: Herbal oils, powders, or juices are administered via the nostrils. *Nasya* effectively controls sinusitis, migraine, and neck stiffness and enhances cognitive functions. It aids in clearing the nasal passages and improves mental clarity.

RAKTAMOKSHANA (BLOOD LETTING THERAPY)

Purpose: To cleanse the blood.

Procedure: Methods such as leech therapy or venepuncture are utilized to expel impure blood. This technique is suggested for issues like skin disorders, varicose veins, gout, and certain types of hypertension. It aids in diminishing inflammation and boosting blood circulation.

PURVA KARMA (PREPARATION PHASE)

SNEHANA (OLEATION)

The internal and external application of medicated oils. Internal oleation involves consuming small quantities of medicated ghee or oil, while external oleation encompasses *Abhyanga* (oil massage). This procedure helps to loosen toxins, making them easier to remove.

SWEDANA (FOMENTATION)

Provoking sweating through steam baths or alternative methods to further loosen toxins. It amplifies the advantages of *Snehana* by opening the pores and aiding the elimination of toxins through sweat.

PRADHANA KARMA (MAIN TREATMENT PHASE)

This phase includes carrying out the five main *Panchakarma* procedures (*Vamana*, *Virechana*, *Basti*, *Nasya*, and *Raktamokshana*) according to the individual's constitution and specific health concerns.

The selection of procedure is tailored to guarantee optimal effectiveness in *Panchakarma* detoxification and *Dosha* balance.

PASCHAT KARMA (POST-TREATMENT PHASE)

Dietary Regimen: A particular diet is suggested to assist the digestive system in recovery and to avert the buildup of new toxins. Light and easily digestible foods are prioritized.

Lifestyle Changes: Patients receive recommendations on lifestyle adjustments, including daily practices, exercise, yoga, and meditation routines to sustain the advantages of detoxification and promote overall well-being.

BENEFITS OF PANCHAKARMA

Panchakarma is a profound and transformative therapy that can bring about significant improvements in overall health and well-being. *Panchakarma*, is a comprehensive detoxification and rejuvenation therapy. There are multiple benefits of *Panchakarma* as below-

- **Detoxification**: By eliminating stored toxins (ama) from the body, Panchakarma improves overall health and prevents disease development. Detoxification enhances the body's natural healing capabilities and increases energy levels.
- **Restores Dosha Balance**: Achieving balance among the three *Doshas (Vata, Pitta,* and *Kapha)* is crucial for sustaining health.

Panchakarma assists in restoring this equilibrium, enhancing bodily functions and mental clarity.

- **Enhances Immunity**: Detoxification and rejuvenation fortify the immune system, making the body more resilient against infections and illnesses. They also improve the body's capacity to combat pathogens.
- **Improves Digestion**: *Panchakarma* stimulates and regulates digestive enzymes and metabolic functions, resulting in improved digestion and nutrient absorption. It addresses digestive problems such as indigestion, bloating, and constipation.
- **Promotes Weight Loss**: *Panchakarma* supports weight management by enhancing metabolism and removing toxins. It helps decrease fat storage and encourages a healthy body weight.
- **Mental Clarity and Emotional Well-being**: *Panchakarma* alleviates stress, anxiety, and depression by detoxifying the body and harmonizing the mind. It fosters mental clarity, emotional stability, and improves cognitive abilities.
- **Skin Health**: Detoxification and nourishment through *Panchakarma* enhance skin tone and wellness. It aids in treating various skin conditions including eczema, psoriasis and acne.

Panchakarma is an impactful Ayurvedic therapy designed to detoxify and rejuvenate the body. By grasping the comprehensive processes and advantages, you can recognize how Panchakarma contributes to maintaining and restoring health. It efficiently eliminates toxins, balances *Doshas*, and improves overall health and wellness.

NASYA KARMA

For the treatment of Suprasternal disease (*Urdhva-jatrugata roga*), *Nasya* is the most important therapy. By using *Panchakarma* procedure not only cure the disease but also prevent the disease. As **Acharya Sushrut** says: -

संचयेऽपहृताः दोषाः लभन्ते नोत्तरा गतिः ।
तेत्तूत्तराषु गतिषु भवन्ति बलवत्तराः ।। सु.सू. 21/37

The preference of knowing the manifestation of a disease at every level is of utmost importance in controlling the disease. The **Acharya Charak** have also said-

द्वारं हि शिरसो नासा। च.सि. 9/89

Because *Nasa* is indirectly connected with the brain centers within the head. *Nasa* is considered to be that *Indriya*, whose function are not only limited to respiration but is also considered as a pathway for drug administration.

Medicine or medicated oil administered through Nasal path is known as *Nasya*.

औषधमौषधसिद्धो वा स्नेहो नासिकाभ्यां दीयते इति नस्यम्। सु.चि. 40/21

According to **Bhavprakash** all drugs and measures that are administered through the Nasal root are known as Nasya. According to **Acharya Sharangdhar**, *Naavan* and *Nasya* are the two name of this therapy. **Arundatta** states *'Nasayam kiyata iti Nasyam'* which clearly indicate the route of administration.

Nasya is a therapeutic measure where the medicated oil, *Kwath, Swarasa, Churna* etc used for elimination the vitiated *Doshas* situated in *Shira* for the treatment of *Urdhvajatrugata Vikara*.

SIGNIFICANCE OF NASYA KARMA

As Ayurvedic ***Acharyas*** said that *'Nasa hi shirso dwaaram'* so all the disease above the clavicle cured by this therapy. *Nasya Karma* has the following benefits:

- Due to presence of highly vascularized mucosa, increased the drug absorption through Nasal passage.
- Improved bioavailability
- Lower side effects

CLASSIFICATION OF *NASYA*

The *Nasya* is five types i.e. *Navana, Avapida, Dhmapana, Dhuma* and *Pratimarsa*. According to pharmacological action, *Nasya* has been classified into three groups i.e. *Rechana, Tarpana* and *Shamana*. According to part of the drugs to be used in *Nasya karma,* **Acharya**

Charak has also mentioned seven types of *Nasya* i.e. *Phala, Patra, Moola, Kanda, Puspa, Niryasa* and *Twak*.

NAVANA NASYA

Navana is one of the important and well applicable therapies of *Nasya Karma*. It can be mainly classified into *Snehana* and *Shodhana*. *Navana* is administered by instilling the drops of a medicated oil or *ghrita* in the nose. According to **Acharya Sushrut**, *Navana* is generally a *Sneha Nasya* and is known as *Nasya* in general.

SNEHANA NASYA

It is used for the feeling of head lightness, it gives strength to neck, shoulder and chest region and beneficial for eyesight.

Dose: The following is the dosage schedule for *Sneha Nasya*.

- *Hina Matra* – 8 drops in each nostril.
- *Madhyama Matra* –16 drops in each nostril *(Shukti Pramana)*
- *Uttama Matra* – 32 drops in each nostril *(Panishukti Pramana)*

Bhoja has mentioned 8 drops for *Prayogika Sneha Nasya* and 16 drops for *Sneihika Nasya*.

SHODHANA NASYA

Shirovirechana can be categorized in *Shodhana* type of *Navana Nasya*. In this type of *Nasya* oil prepared by *Shirovirechaka dravya* like *Vidanga, Apamarga, Shigru* etc. can be used.

Dose: According to *Sushrut*, it can be given in following dosage schedule-

- *Uttama* - 8 drops
- *Madhyama* - 6 drops
- *Hina* - 4 drops

TIME OF ADMINISTRATION OF NASYA

Navana Nasya should be administered according to the following time schedule.

- In *Kaphaja Roga:* Fore noon (*Purvahan*)
- In *Pittaja Roga*: Noon (*Madhyahan*)
- In *Vataja Roga*: After Noon (*Aparahan*)

Ashtang Hridaya described time schedule of *Nasya* in healthy persons as follows.

- *Sheeta Kala*: Noon (*Madhyahane*)
- *Sharada* and *Vasanta*: Fore Noon (*Purvahane*)
- *Grishma Ritu*: Evening (*Aparahane*)
- *Varsha Ritu*: During the presence of Sunlight (*Aatape*)

AVAPIDA NASYA

अवपीड्य यत्र कल्कादीनि दीयन्ते इत्यवपीडः। च.सि. 9/90 चक्रपाणि

The word *Avapida Nasya* means *Nasya* given by extracted juice of leaves or pest (*kalk*) of required medicine. *Avapida Nasya* is from *kalkadi* (*Kalka,Kwatha,Swarasa* etc.) It is *tikshna murdha Rechana* and is a strong purgative to head. It is of two types.

1. *Stambhana Nasya*
2. *Shodhana Nasya*

DOSE OF AVAPIDA NASYA

The dosage of *Avapida Nasya* is as like as *Shirovirechana* viz, 4, 6, 8 drops is *Hina, Madhyama* and *Uttama Matra* respectively.

DHMAPANA NASYA

Dhmapana Nasya is a variety of *Shodhana Nasya*. It is also known as *Pradhamana Nasya*. The *Churna* is administered through nasal passage with the help of *Nadi Yantra*, which is *6 Angula* long and both sides open ended. The *Churna* of required drug is kept at one end and air is blown from the other end so that medicine may enter into the nostrils. **Videha** has mentioned another method for *Pradhamana*. In which fine powder of drug kept in a *Pottali* made by a thin cloth is used to inhale so that smallest particles of the medicine enter into the nostrils.

INDICATION

चेतोविकारकृमिविषाभिपन्नानां चूर्णं प्रधमेत्। सु.चि. 40/46

Chetovikara, Krimija Shiroroga, Vishabhipanna.

Dose: According to Videha the dose of *Dhmapana Nasya* is three *Muchuti* (3 pinch). For the *Pottali* method *Churna* should be *Shukti Pramana.*

DHUMA NASYA

Dhuma Nasya is defined as medicated fume taken by nasal passage and eliminated by oral route. According to **Chakrapani**, fume taken by mouth is known as *Dhumapana* and is not included in *Nasya. Dhuma Nasya is of 3 types. i.e. Prayogika, Snehika, and Vairechanika.* **Acharya Charak** has mentioned *Dhuma Nadi* for *Dhuma Nasya.*

The breadth of *Dhuma Nadi* is of measuring one's own finger and length for *Virechana* type 24 *Angula*, for *Snehika Dhuma* 32 *Angula* length, for *Prayogika Dhuma* 36 *Angula* is suggested.

DOSE OF PRAYOGIKA DHUMA

During the prescribed times, a wise person should smoke twice for *Prayogika Dhuma* (habitual variety). Once for *Snehika Dhuma* (unctuous variety). And three to four times for the *Virechanic Dhuma* (eliminative variety). For *Prayogika Dhuma* drugs like *Harenuka, Priyangu, Ushira* etc. should be used. For *Snehika Dhuma*, *Vasa, Ghrita* etc. and for *Virechanic Dhuma,* drugs like *Aparajita, Apamarga* etc. should be used.

PRATIMARSHA NASYA

प्रतिमर्शस्तु नस्यार्थं करोति न च दोषवान् ।
नस्तः स्नेहांगुलि दद्यात् प्रातनिशि च सर्वदा।। च.सि. 9/117

Pratimarsha Nasya is given by dipping the finger in the required *Sneha* and then dropping it in the nostrils and it does not aggravate the *Doshas*. It could be given daily and even in all the seasons in morning and evening.

DOSE OF PRATIMARSHA NASYA

ईषदुच्छिंघनात् स्नेहो यावान् वक्त्रं प्रपद्यते ।
नस्तो निषिक्तं तं विद्यात् प्रतिमर्शं प्रमाणतः।। च.सि.9/117 चक्रपाणि

Chakrapani described that when the patient sneezes a little amount of *Sneha* goes to mouth, the *Sneha Nasya* given in this dose is said as the dose of *Pratimarsa Nasya*. Two drops in each nostril at morning and evening. The Sneha should at least reach from *Nasa* to *kantha* but it should not be too much that could produce secretion in *Kantha* (throat).

INDICATION

Pratimarsha could be given daily, in any age, and even in all the seasons at morning and evening. i.e.

- *Varsha*
- *Bala & Vriddha*

- *Durdina*
- *Kshata*
- *Sukhatma*

Acharya Sushrut and **Sharangdhara** have described 14 suitable times for *Pratimarsha Nasya*, while **Vagbhat** has mentioned 15 *Kaal.*

MARSHA NASYA

According to **Vagbhat** dropping 6-10 drops of *Sneha* in the nostrils is known as *marsha nasya*. *Pratimarsha* and *Marsha* are same in principle, but the main difference between them is *matra*.

DOSE OF MARSHA NASYA

In Marsha nasya, 6-10 *bindu* of *sneha* is used. All *snehna dravyas* like *taila, gritha* etc can be used, but use of *taila* is more applicable due to its *Kapha hara* properties and *shira* being the *Kapha sthana*.

MARSHA-PRATIMARSHA NASYA

Marsha and *Pratimarsha* both consist of introduction of oils through the nostrils. It is well tolerated and is very much convenient procedure. Both of the *Nasya* are same in principles, but the main difference between them is of dose. On the basis of their doses **Acharya Vagbhat** has classified *Sneha Nasya* into *Pratimarsha* and *Marsha*. This *Nasya* causes no *Vyapat* and it's safe.

INDICATIONS OF NASYA

Acharya Charak has described the following general indications where *Nasya* therapy should be used.

Shirastambha	Skandha Roga
Dantastambha	Amsashoola
Manyastambha	Nasikaroga
Galagraha	Akshiroga
Hanugraha	Karna Roga
Pinasa	Shira Kapala Roga
Galashundika	Shiroroga Ardita
Kantha Saluki	Apatantraka
Sukra Roga	Apatanaka
Timira Roga	Arbuda
Vartma Roga	Swarbheda
Vyanga	Vakgraha
Upajihvika	Gadgadatva
Ardhavbhedaka	Grivaroga

CONTRAINDICATIONS OF NASYA

In *Ayurvedic* classics, some special conditions have been mentioned in which *Nasya* should not be administered, otherwise various complications may occur. *Nasya* should not be administered on *durdina* (rainy day), this is a general rule but it is also said that in emergency condition seasonal regime can be over ruled.

SUITABLE TIME FOR GIVING NASYA

प्रावृटशरद्वसन्तेतरेष्वात्ययिकेषु रोगेषु नावनं कुर्यात् कृत्रिमगुणोपधानात्, ग्रीष्मे पूर्वाह्ने, शीते मध्याह्ने, वर्षास्वदुर्दिने चेति।। च.सि. 2/23

According to **Charak** generally *Nasya* should be given in *Pravrita, Sharada* and *Vasant Ritu*. However, in emergency it can be given in any season by providing artificial conditions of the above-mentioned seasons. It should be given in *Grishma Ritu* before noon (morning), *Sheeta Ritu* in noon and in *Varsha Ritu* when day should be clear.

According to **Sushrut** in normal conditions *Nasya* should be given in empty stomach, at the time when the person usually takes his meal. He also advised time schedule in *Doshaja vikara* as follows-

Doshaja Vikara	Nasya Administration Time
Kaphaja Vikara	Morning
Pittaja Vikara	Noon
Vataja Vikara	Evening

COURSE OF NASYA KARMA

- **CHARAK** has mentioned specific duration of the *Nasya* therapy, in context of *Anu tail. Nasya* can be given on alternate day-thrice daily for seven days.

- **SUSHRUT** -*Nasya* can be given repeatedly at the interval of 1, 2, 7 and 21 days depending upon the condition of the patient and the disease.
- **VAGBHAT -** *Nasya Karma* may be given for seven consecutive days. In conditions like *Vata Dosha* in head, hiccough, torticollis, loss of voice etc. it may be done twice a day (in morning and evening).

DOSE OF NASYA KARMA

The dose of *Nasya* drug depends upon the drug utilized for it and the variety of the therapy. **Charak** has not prescribed the dose of the *Nasya*. **Sushrut** and **Vagbhat** have mentioned the dose in the form of *Bindus* (drops), here one *Bindu* means the drop which is formed after dipping the two phalanges of *Pradeshini* (index) finger.

ADMINISTRATION OF NASYA

The procedure of giving *Nasya* therapy may be classified into the following three headings-

- *Purvakarma* (Pre-measures)
- *Pradhanakarma* (Nasya Therapy)
- *Paschatkarma* (Post measures)

Table: Dose of Nasya in Bindu for each nostril

Sl. No.	Type of Nasya	Drops in each Nostril		
		Hrasva Matra	Madhyama Matra	Uttam Matra
1	Shamana Nasya	8	16	32
2	Shodhana Nasya	4	6	8
3	Marsha Nasya	6	8	10
4	Avapida Nasya	4	6	8
5	Pratimarsha Nasya	2	2	2

PURVAKARMA OF NASYA THERAPY

1. COLLECTION OF NECESSARY MATERIALS:

Before giving *Nasya*, prior arrangement of the material and equipment's should be done. There should be a special room "*Nasya Bhavana*" free from atmospheric effects like direct blow of air and dust, etc. and with appropriate light arrangement. Following articles should be collected before *Nasya*: -

NASYA ASANA

(a) A chair for sitting, (b) A cot for lying.

Drugs required for *shirovirechana* should be collected in the form of *kalka, churna, kwatha, kshira, udaka, sneha, asava, dhuma* etc. in sufficient quantity.

NASYA YANTRA

For *Snehana*, *Avapida*, *Marsha* and *Pratimarsha Nasya*, there should be a dropper or *Pichu*. For *Pradhamana Nasya shadangula nadi* and specific *dhumayantra* for *Dhum Nasya* are required.

SELECTION OF THE PATIENT

The patient should be selected according to the indications and contraindications of *Nasya* described in classics. For *Nasya Karma*, suitable age of patient must be in between 7 to 80 yrs.

PREPARATION OF PATIENT

- The patient should pass the natural urges like urine, stool etc.
- **Abhyang (Massage)**: The patient advice to lie down on *Nasya* table. *Mridu Abhyanga* should be done on scalp, forehead, face and neck for 5-10 minutes by medicated oil like *Tila Taila* etc.
- **Swedana (Suddation)**: According to Ayurvedic classics *swedana* should not be given to the head. *Mridu swedana* should be given for elimination of *Doshas* and liquification of *Doshas*.
- For *Mridu swedana Panitapa sweda* (fomented by warm palm) or cloth dipped in hot water should be given on scalp, forehead, face and neck.

PRADHANA KARMA OF NASYA THERAPY

As described by **Charak** (Ch.Si. 9/98-99), **Vagbhat** (A.H.Su. 20/18-20) and **Sushrut** (Su.Chi. 40/25-27) the following procedure should be adopted for performing the *Nasya Karma.*

- Patient should lie down in supine position with ease on *Nasya* table.
- *Shira* (head) should be "*Pralambita*" (lowering or head down position) and feet slightly raised. Head should not be excessively flexed or extended.
- If the head is not lowered, the nasal medication may not reach to the desired distinction and if it is lowered too much, there may be the danger of getting the medication to be lodged in brain.
- After covering the eyes with clean cotton cloth, the physician should raise the tip of the patient's nose with his left thumb and with the right hand the luke warm medicine (*Sukhoshna* drug) should be dropped in both the nostrils alternately in proper way.
- The drug should be neither less nor more in the dose i.e. it should be in the proper quantity.
- It should also be neither very hot nor very cold. i.e. it should be Luke warm.
- The patient should avoid speech, anger, sneezing, laughing and head shaking during *Nasya Karma*.

SAMYAKA YOGA, AYOGA AND ATIYOGA OF NASYA

After *Nasya Karma* the symptoms of its *Samyaka Yoga, Ayoga* and *Atiyoga* should be observed which are being described here under.

SAMYAKA YOGA

उरःशिरोलाघवमिन्द्रियाच्छयं स्रोतोविशुद्धिश्च भवेद्विशुद्धेः । च.सि. 1/51

The symptoms of adequate *Nasya* according to **Charak** are *urah-shiro-laghava* (Feeling of lightness in chest and head), *indriyavishuddhi* (sensorial proficiency) and *srotovishuddhi* (cleansing of channels).

लाघवं शिरसः शुद्धिः स्रोतसां व्याधिनिर्णयः ।
चित्तेन्द्रियप्रसादश्च शिरसः शुद्धिलक्षणम् ।। सु.चि. 40/38

Sushrut has described *shira laghuta* (lightness in head), *chitta indriya prasadana* (mental and sensorial happiness) and *vikaropashama* (improvement).

सम्यक् स्निग्धे सुखेच्छ्वासस्वप्नबोधाक्षपाटवम् । अ.हृ.सू. 20/23

Besides this proper respiration, sound sleep & wake up at time and *indriya suddhi* have been described by **Vagbhat** as the general symptoms of *samyak yoga* of *Nasya Karma.*

AYOGA

गलोपलेपः शिरसो गुरूत्वं निष्ठीवनं चाप्यथ दुर्विरिक्ते । च.सि. 1/52

If *Nasya* is not given in proper way or the dose is less, features of inadequate *Nasya* occur which are *galopalepa* (throat coated with mucus), *shirogaurava* (heaviness in head) and *nishthivana* (excessive spitting).

कण्डूपदेहौ गुरुता स्रोतसां कफसंस्रवः ।
मूर्ध्नि हीनविशुद्धे तु लक्षणं परिकीर्तितम् ।। सु.चि. 40/39

According to Sushrut, *kandu* (itching in nose), *upadeha* (feeling of wetness), *guruta* (heaviness), *Srotasam Kapha srava* (excess mucus secretion in channesl) are the symptoms of *hina shuddhi*.

रूक्षेऽक्षिस्तब्धता शोषो नासास्ये मूर्द्धशून्यता। अ.हृ.सू. 20/24

Vitiation of *Vata,* dryness in *indriya* and no relief in the symptoms of the diseases; dryness in mouth and nose are also the symptoms of *Ayoga* of *Nasya Karma*.

ATIYOGA

शिरोऽक्षिशंखश्रवणार्तितोदावत्यर्थशुद्धे तिमिरं च पश्येत्। च.सि. 1/52

According to **Charak**, the general features of excessive *Nasya* are feeling of *Arati* (uneasiness) and *Toda* (pricking like pain in the head, eyes, temporal region and ears).

कफप्रसेकः शिरसो गुरुतेन्द्रियविभ्रमः। सु.चि. 40/34

Kapha srava (salivation), *shirahshoola* (headache) and *indriya vibhrama* (confusion) are the other symptoms of *Atiyoga* of *Nasya*.

मस्तुलुंगागमोः वातवृद्धिरिन्द्रियविभ्रमः ।
शून्यता शिरसश्चापि मूर्ध्नि गाढविरेचिते।। सु.चि. 40/40

Mastulungagama, Vata Vriddhi, indriyavibhrama and *shiroshunyata* (emptiness of head) are also the symptoms of *Atiyoga* of *Shirovirechana*.

स्निग्धेऽतिकण्डूगुरुताप्रसेकारुचिपीनसाः । अ.हृ.सू. 20/24

Kandu (itching), *guruta* (feeling of heaviness of the head), *praseka* (excess salivation), *aruchi* (anorexia), *peenasa* (rhinitis) are signs of *Atiyoga* of *Sneha Nasya*.

VYAPADA (COMPLICATIONS) OF NASYA

The patients after taking the *Nasya Karma* if does not follow the regimen given above then the *Prakopa* of ***Dosha*** may again occur leading to many complications which are known as *Vyapada*.

Many complications of *Nasya Karma* may occur due to administration of *Nasya* when it is contraindicated and due to technical failure.

दोषोत्क्लेशनिमित्तास्तु जयेच्छमनशोधनैः ।
अथ क्षयनिमित्तासु यथास्वं बृंहणं हितम् ।। सु.चि. 40/50

These complications occur through following two modes. (a) *Doshotklesh* which can be managed by *Shodhana* and *Shamana Chikitsa* and (b) *Dosha Kshaya* which has to be managed by *Brimhana Chikitsa*.

If *Nasya* is given in the contraindicated conditions like *Ajirna, Bhuktabhakta, Jalapita, Nava Pratisyaya* etc. or in season or time where *Nasya karma* is contraindicated e.g. cloudy atmosphere, then there is possibility of production of *Kapha rogas* like *swasa, kasa* etc. In such conditions, the treatment should be done with *Kapha Nashaka Upachara* like use of *Ushna* and *Tikshna Aushadha* and *Karma*.

If *Nasya* is given in *Krishasharira* (emaciated), *Virikta* (patient who had taken virechana), *Garbhini* (pregnant lady), *Vyayama klanta* (exhausted with exercise) and in thirsty person then vitiation of *Vata* takes place and may lead to *Vataja Vikara*. In all the above conditions, *Vata Nashak* procedures like *Snehana, Brimhana* and *Swedana* should be done. The pregnant lady should specifically be treated with the use of *Ghrita* and milk.

PASCHAT KARMA

As described by **Charak** (*Ch.Si.* 9/103-107) **Ashtanga Hridaya** (*As.H.Su.* 20/22-23) and **Sushrut** (*Su.Chi.* 40/29-31) following regimen should be followed.

After administration of medication through nasal passage patient should lie supine for about 2-minute time interval & ask him to count numbers up to 100. After an administration of *Nasya,* feet, shoulders, palms and ears should be massaged. The head, cheek and neck should be again subjected to sudation. If possible, snuffing of *Rasna Churna* for *Vata Prashamana* should be done.

- The patient should avoid swallowing of *Nasya Aushadhi* and *Kaphadi Doshas*.
- The oil that has been dropped in the nose may be repeatedly drained out together with the morbid *Doshas*, especially mucus; should be eliminated by the patient by sneezing slowly.
- Care should be taken that not even the smallest portion of the medicated oil should be left behind.
- Patient should spit out the excessive medicine which has come into the oropharynx.
- Medicated *Dhumapana* and *Gandusha* are advocated to expel out the residue mucus lodged in *Kantha* (gullet) and *Shringataka.*
- Patient should stay at windless place. Light meal (*Laghu Aahara*) and luke warm water *(Sukhoshna Jala)* is allowed.

One should avoid dust, smoke, sunshine, alcohol, cold bath, riding, anger, excess fat and liquid diet. Day sleep and cold water for any purpose like *Pana, Snana* etc. should be avoided after *Nasya Karma*.

MODE OF ACTION OF NASYA KARMA

The clear description regarding the mode of action of the *Nasya Karma* is not available in Ayurvedic classics. According to **Charak**, *Nasa* is the gate way of *Shira*. The drug administered through nose as *Nasya* reaches the brain & eliminates only the morbid *Doshas* responsible for producing the disease.

नासा हि शिरसो द्वारं तत्रावसेचितमौषधं स्रोतः श्रृंगाटकं प्राप्य च मूर्धानं नेत्रश्रोत्रकण्ठादिसिरामुखानि च मुंजादिषीकामिवासक्तामूर्धजत्रुगतां वैकारिकीमशेषामाशु दोषसंहतिमुत्तमांगादपकर्षति ।। अ.सं.सू. 29/3

In **Ashtanga Samgraha**, it is explained that *Nasa* being the door way to *shira* (head), the drug administered through nostrils, reaches *Shringataka* (a *Sira Marma* by *Nasa Srota*) and spreads in the *Murdha* (brain) taking route of *Netra* (eye), *Shrota* (ear), *Kantha* (throat), *Siramukhas* (opening of the vessels) etc. and scratches the morbid *Doshas* in supra clavicular region and extracts them from the *Uttamanga*.

Sushrut has clarified *Shringataka Marma* as a *Sira Marma* formed by the union of *Siras* (blood vessels) supplying to nose, ear, eye & tongue. He further points out that injury to this *Marma* will be immediately fatal.

According to all prominent Acharyas, Nasa is said to be the gateway of Shira. It does not mean that any channel connects directly to the brain but they might be connected through blood vessels or through nervous system (olfactory nerve, etc.)

It is an experimentally proven fact that where any type of irritation takes place in any part of the body, the local blood circulation is always increased. This is the result of natural protection function of the body. Something happens when provocation of *Doshas* takes place in *Shira* due to irritating effect of administered drug, which resulting an increase of the blood circulation of brain. So extra accumulated morbid *Dosha* are expelled out from small blood vessels and ultimately these morbid *Doshas* are thrown out by the nasal discharge, tears and by salivation.

MODERN POINT OF VIEW

- There is no such direct Pharmacodynamic consideration between nose & no such cranial organs. Moreover blood-brain barrier in the human body is a strict security system.
- The nose is used as a route of administration for inhalation of anaesthetic materials. In the case of paranasal sinusitis certain agents used as decongestants.
- Since quite a time anterior pituitary hormone, nasal spray is in practice with modern medical system. Vasopressin or Antidiuretic hormone is already in the market in the form of nasal therapy.
- Nasal administrations of luteinising hormone & calcitonin are found to be equally effective as intravenous infusions in maintaining blood concentrations.
- It was claimed that the concentration of drug in C.S.F. was very high to that when administered intravenously.
- Scientists of the institute of medical sciences Delhi have proved after experiments that drug administered through *Nasa* shows

effective action in the brain. So, it can be said that there is a very close relation between *Shira* & *Nasa*.

EFFECT ON DRUGS ABSORPTION

- Keeping the head in lowered position & retention of medicine in naso-pharynx, helps in providing sufficient time for local drug absorption.
- Any liquid soluble substance has greater chance for passive absorption directly through the cells of lining membrane.
- On the other hand, massage & local fomentation also enhances the drug absorption.
- The later course of drug transversion can occur in two ways – by general systemic circulation and by direct pooling into the intracranial region.
- The second way is more of interest in our present study. This direct transportation can be assumed again in two paths, viz. Vascular path & Lymphatic path.

VASCULAR PATH TRANSPORTATION

Vascular Path transportation is possible through the pooling of nasal Venous blood to the facial vein, which naturally occurs. Just of the opposite entrance the inferior ophthalmic veins also pool into the facial vein. Interestingly, both facial and ophthalmic veins have no veinal valves in between. So that, blood may drain on either side, that is to say the blood from facial vein can enter cavernous venous sinus of the brain in reverse direction. Thus, such a pooling of blood from nasal veins to venous sinuses of the brain is more likely in the head lowered position due to gravity. On this line, the absorption of drug materials into meninges and related parts of intracranial organs is worth considering point.

Pooling of blood from paranasal sinuses also possible in the same manner. **Vagbhat's** notation of *Shringataka Srotas* (anterior cranial fossa) seems to relation with the above explanation.

LYMPHATIC PATH TRANSPORTATION

Drug transportation by lymphatic path, can reach direct into the C.S.F. It is known that the arachnoid matter sleeve is extended to the submucosal area of the nose along with olfactory nerve. Experiments have shown that the dye injected to arachnoid matter has caused coloration of nasal mucosa within seconds and vice versa also.

Here it may be worthy to recall Sushrut's caution that the excessive administration of *Virechana Nasya* (eliminative errhine) may cause oozing of *Mastulunga* (C.S.F.) into the nose. On this basis, we may say that ancient scholars of **Ayurveda** were aware of the lymphatic path in direct absorption into the brain from nose.

IMPORTANCE OF POST NASYA MASSAGE

The Ayurvedic texts recommended light massage on the frontal, temporal, maxillary, mastoid and on *Manya* region. A comfortable massage on the above region may help to subside the irritation of somatic construction due to heat stimulation. It may also help in removing the slush created in these regions. However, interesting here is regarding *Manya* which is a *Marma* existing in neck on either side of the trachea which likely correspond to the carotid sinuses of the neck. Pressure applied on the baroreceptors may bring the deranged cerebral arterial pressure to normalcy. Because these receptors lying on bed of bifurcation of common carotid artery have a buffering action on the cerebral arterial pressure.

On the basis of the foregoing observations, we can state that the procedures, postures & conducts explained for *Nasya Karma* are of vital importance in drug absorption & transportation.

- $$$ -

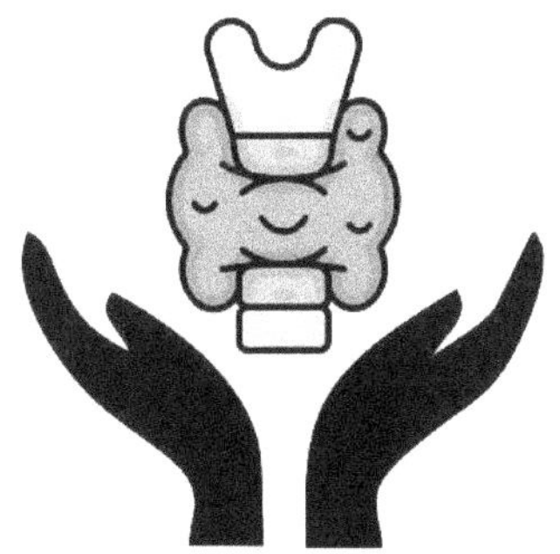

Drugs for Thyroid Disorders

Dr. Ajay Kumar, Dr. Tina Singhal

The hormones produced by the thyroid gland are released into the bloodstream and distributed to all body tissues. Thyroid hormones have a significant impact on growth, development, and the control of metabolism. Several factors can impact the levels of these hormones, and the well-being of the thyroid relies on numerous genetic, dietary, and immune-related factors that can result in either over or underactivity. Various herbs have been demonstrated to support thyroid function by utilizing distinct mechanisms tailored to the body's requirements. Utilizing herbal adaptogens, anti-inflammatories, & immunomodulators is frequently a crucial component of a holistic strategy to aid in maintaining optimal thyroid function.

Managing hypothyroidism typically necessitates a comprehensive, individualized approach and a deep comprehension of the particular imbalance or pathology. The typical approach for treating thyroid problems is through hormone replacement therapy, whether it is synthetic or desiccated. While this therapy may work well for certain individuals, others may find that solely using thyroid hormone does not treat the root cause of the problem or alleviate their symptoms. Herbal approaches, along with dietary and lifestyle changes, have been successfully utilized in traditional medical models to treat thyroid dysfunction. Some herbal agents are currently being investigated for their effectiveness in hypothyroidism, hyperthyroidism, and autoimmune diseases, showing positive outcomes in preclinical and clinical research.

Ayurvedic classics give importance to *Aushadha* as a part of *Trisutra Ayurveda.* Selection of drug for *Chikitsa* depends chiefly on pathological factors *(Samprapti Ghataka),* disease itself, and cardinal features etc. Modern medical science treats Hypothyroidism with the hormonal pill i.e. Levothyroxine. This is a one type of supplementary therapy.

The substance or any product having rasa or extract which is used for treatment of disease of a patient and maintain the health of a healthy person is known as *Aushadhi.* Various drugs are suggesting its importance next to physician. From the Ayurvedic point of view, *Kapha Dosha* plays a major role in the pathogenesis of hypothyroidism as most of the symptoms present in it are due to vitiation of *Kapha*

Dosha. Secondary vitiation of *Vata Dosha* is also present in it. In this disease condition, the function of *Pitta Dosha* is found below to its normal level.

According to **Acharya Bhav Prakash,** *Galagand*, *Gandamala*, *Granthi*, *Apchi*, *Arbud Adhikar Chikitsa* has stated to use its *Kanchnar twak kwath* with *Shunthi churna* & *Nimb tail Nasya* by **Acharya Chakradatt**, has given in the chapter of *Galgand, Gandmala, Apchi Granthi Arbud Adhikar Chikitsa*

KANCHNAR

Kanchnar or Bauhinia variegata, also known as mountain ebony or orchid tree, has shown potential effects on the thyroid gland due to its bioactive compounds like flavonoids, alkaloids, tannins, and saponins.

Bauhinia variegata shows promise in managing thyroid conditions, particularly hyperthyroidism, due to its anti-thyroid and antioxidant properties.

Here's a detailed point-wise summary of its potential effects:

IMPROVED THYROID HORMONE LEVELS

- Studies on animals show that Bauhinia variegata extract can increase levels of T3 and T4, the key hormones produced by the thyroid gland. It can also reduce TSH levels, a hormone that's often elevated in hypothyroidism.

COMBINED THERAPY POTENTIAL

- Research suggests that using Bauhinia variegata with *Commiphora mukul* might have a more significant impact than using either herb individually. One study published in the "Journal of Drug Delivery and Therapeutics" (2019) investigated the effects of Bauhinia variegata and *Commiphora mukul* extracts on methimazole-induced hypothyroidism in rats. The study found that a combination of high doses of both plant extracts significantly lowered TSH levels.
- Another study in the "Journal of Pharmacognosy and Phytochemistry" (2019) also used a rat model of methimazole-induced hypothyroidism and found that combined extracts of *Bauhinia variegata* and *Commiphora mukul* had more beneficial effects on thyroid function than individual plant extracts.

ENHANCED THYROID GLAND HEALTH

- Animal studies have indicated that Bauhinia variegata can improve thyroid gland histology.

ANTIOXIDANT EFFECTS

- Bauhinia variegata is a source of antioxidants, specifically flavonoids, which can help protect the thyroid gland from damage. Oxidative stress can impair thyroid function.
- *Bauhinia variegata* also contains saponins, which may influence

hormone production and have anti-inflammatory effects.

- Other phytochemicals in *Bauhinia variegata*, such as tannins and alkaloids, may also contribute to its therapeutic effects on thyroid function through various mechanisms.

PRECAUTIONS

- **Limited Human Studies:** More research, especially clinical trials involving humans, is needed to confirm *Bauhinia variegata's* efficacy and safety for managing hypothyroidism in humans.
- Limited clinical trials have evaluated the effects of *Bauhinia variegata* on thyroid function in humans.
- **Mechanisms of Action:** The exact ways in which *Bauhinia variegata* affects thyroid function are not fully understood. Some proposed mechanisms include modulating thyroid hormone production, antioxidant activity, anti-inflammatory effects, and modulation of the HPT axis.
- The antioxidant properties of *Bauhinia variegata* may protect the thyroid gland from oxidative damage, which can impair thyroid function.
- Chronic inflammation can contribute to thyroid dysfunction, and *Bauhinia variegata's* anti-inflammatory properties may help alleviate this.
- Additionally, *Bauhinia variegata* may influence the feedback

mechanisms within the HPT axis, leading to changes in TSH and thyroid hormone levels.

SAFETY AND POTENTIAL SIDE EFFECTS

- *Bauhinia variegata* is generally considered safe for consumption in moderate amounts. However, some people might experience mild side effects such as gastrointestinal issues or allergic reactions.

DRUG INTERACTIONS

- It is important to be aware of potential drug interactions with *Bauhinia variegata*, especially if taking medications for thyroid disorders, diabetes, or other chronic conditions.
- Pregnant or breastfeeding women and individuals with underlying medical conditions should consult with a healthcare professional before using *Bauhinia variegata*.

SHUNTHI

It consists of dried rhizome of *Zingiber Officinale* Roxb. (Fam. Zingiberaceae), widely cultivated in India, rhizomes dug in January-February, buds and roots removed, soaked overnight-in water, decorticated, and sometimes treated with lime and dried. Zingiber officinale (*Ginger*) is a medicinal plant with potential benefits for thyroid health due to its antioxidant, anti-inflammatory, and lipid-modulating effects. However, more clinical studies are needed to confirm its efficacy, especially in regards to thyroid disorders.

Here's a detailed summary of its potential benefits:

ANTIOXIDANT EFFECTS

- Ginger contains potent antioxidants like gingerols, shogaols, and zingerone.
- These compounds neutralize free radicals and protect thyroid cells from oxidative damage.
- This may be beneficial for autoimmune thyroid conditions like Hashimoto's thyroiditis and Graves' disease.

ANTI-INFLAMMATORY EFFECTS

- Gingerols and shogaols inhibit inflammatory mediators, including prostaglandins, cytokines, and leukotrienes, which may reduce thyroid inflammation.
- This may be beneficial for conditions like subacute thyroiditis or autoimmune thyroiditis.

EFFECTS ON THYROID HORMONES

- **Hyperthyroidism**: Ginger may help alleviate symptoms of oxidative stress caused by high thyroid hormone levels. However, its direct role in reducing hormone production is unclear.
- **Hypothyroidism**: Ginger may indirectly support thyroid function

by enhancing metabolism, reducing inflammation, and improving lipid profiles. Its direct effect on T3, T4, or TSH levels in humans needs more research.

- Animal studies suggest ginger may modulate the hypothalamic-pituitary-thyroid (HPT) axis, which regulates thyroid hormone production.

LIPID PROFILE AND CARDIOVASCULAR HEALTH

- Ginger improves lipid metabolism and can reduce total cholesterol, LDL cholesterol, and triglycerides while raising HDL cholesterol.
- This effect may benefit hypothyroid patients prone to dyslipidaemia and cardiovascular risks.

WEIGHT AND METABOLISM

- Ginger supports metabolism and energy expenditure, which could benefit those with hypothyroidism who experience weight gain.

POTENTIAL INTERACTIONS

- Ginger may interact with thyroid hormone replacement drugs (e.g., levothyroxine) or antithyroid medications.
- It is important to separate the timing of ginger consumption and thyroid medication to avoid potential interactions.

While ginger shows promise as a complementary therapy for thyroid health, more clinical studies are needed to confirm its efficacy and mechanism of action in thyroid disorders. It's important to consult a healthcare provider before using ginger to avoid potential interactions with medications or symptom exacerbation.

NIMBA

Nimba consists of whole dried fruit including seeds of *Azadirachta indica* A. Juss. syn. *Melia azadirachta Linn.* (Fam. Meliaceae). Neem is a medicinal plant that has been studied for its potential effects on the thyroid gland. Research, primarily conducted on animals, suggests that neem possesses properties that could influence thyroid hormone levels and overall gland function. Here's a detailed point-wise summary:

HYPOTHYROID EFFECTS:

- Neem exhibits properties that may reduce thyroid hormone levels in the body. Studies indicate that neem extracts might inhibit thyroid peroxidase (TPO), an enzyme crucial for thyroid hormone synthesis.
- Animal studies have demonstrated that neem leaf extract administration lowers serum T3 (triiodothyronine) and T4 (thyroxine) levels, suggesting a direct hypothyroid effect.
- One study showed that rats treated with neem leaf extract for

several weeks had a significant decrease in thyroid hormone levels, indicating the potential of neem to suppress thyroid function at certain doses.

- Prolonged use of neem or high doses could exacerbate hypothyroidism.

ANTIOXIDANT AND ANTI-INFLAMMATORY EFFECTS

- Neem contains bioactive compounds like *quercetin*, *nimbin*, and *azadirachtin* that have antioxidant and anti-inflammatory properties.
- Oxidative stress can negatively impact thyroid gland function, contributing to disorders like hypothyroidism or autoimmune thyroiditis. Neem's antioxidant effects could protect thyroid tissues from oxidative damage.
- Neem's anti-inflammatory action may benefit chronic thyroid inflammation (e.g., Hashimoto's thyroiditis), potentially mitigating the progression of thyroid dysfunction.

POTENTIAL MECHANISMS OF ACTION

Neem's hypothyroid effects are thought to occur through several mechanisms:

- Inhibition of the hypothalamic-pituitary-thyroid (HPT) axis, which regulates thyroid hormone production.
- Modulation of deiodinase enzymes, which convert T4 to the more

active T3, further lowering T3 levels.

- Cytotoxic effects on thyroid cells at high doses, potentially contributing to decreased hormone output.

Given its hypothyroid activity, neem may have potential applications in:

- **Hyperthyroidism**: As an adjunct therapy to help reduce excessive thyroid hormone production.
- **Thyroid Protection**: Its antioxidant properties could support thyroid health in oxidative stress-related conditions.

RISKS AND PRECAUTIONS

- While neem's thyroid-suppressing effects could be beneficial in hyperthyroidism, they pose risks for hypothyroid individuals.
- Neem might interact with thyroid medications, altering their effectiveness.
- Neem has been linked to effects on reproductive hormones, which can indirectly influence thyroid function.
- Neem should be used under medical guidance, particularly in individuals with pre-existing thyroid conditions.

Neem demonstrates potential in managing thyroid conditions, particularly hyperthyroidism, due to its hypothyroid and antioxidant properties. However, its potential to suppress thyroid hormone synthesis necessitates cautious use, especially in hypothyroid individuals. Consulting a healthcare professional before using neem for thyroid health or any other condition is crucial to ensure safety and efficacy.

ASHWAGANDHA

Ashwagandha, also known as *Withania somifera*, is a renowned adaptogen utilized in Ayurvedic practices & is famous for its strong abilities to modulate the immune system and reduce inflammation. Animal's studies of *withania* have demonstrated positive effects on the thyroid gland. One participant with subclinical hypothyroidism saw their condition improve after eight weeks of treatment with Ashwagandha. Every individual who received treatment with Ashwagandha experienced a rise in T4 levels when compared to their initial baseline.

In a recent study, Ashwagandha was shown to help improve thyroid function in patients with subclinical hypothyroidism. However, caution may be needed in cases of hyperthyroidism due to one reported incident of increased thyroxine levels while taking Ashwagandha. Here's a detailed point-wise summary of Ashwagandha's effects on the thyroid:

EFFECTS ON HYPOTHYROIDISM

- **Stimulation of Thyroid Hormones**: Ashwagandha may increase the production of T3 and T4 hormones, potentially improving symptoms of hypothyroidism.

- **Improved Metabolism**: By increasing T3 and T4 levels, Ashwagandha can enhance metabolic rate and energy production, countering the sluggishness often associated with hypothyroidism.
- **Regulation of TSH**: Some evidence suggests that Ashwagandha can help normalize thyroid-stimulating hormone (TSH) levels, balancing overall thyroid function.
- **Clinical Studies**: Clinical trials have shown Ashwagandha supplementation can improve TSH, T3, and T4 levels in individuals with subclinical hypothyroidism. A 2018 study published in the *Journal of Alternative and Complementary Medicine* found that Ashwagandha root extract improved these hormone levels in individuals with subclinical hypothyroidism.

MECHANISMS OF ACTION

- **Adaptogenic Properties**: Helps the body adapt to stress, which can indirectly support thyroid health, as chronic stress is a known contributor to thyroid dysfunction.
- **Antioxidant Activity**: Reduces oxidative stress in thyroid tissues, protecting them from damage and improving function.
- **Hypothalamic-Pituitary-Thyroid Axis Regulation**: Modulates the feedback loop responsible for thyroid hormone production and regulation.

- **Stress Reduction and HPA Axis Modulation**: Ashwagandha's adaptogenic properties help regulate cortisol levels and restore balance to the HPT axis, indirectly supporting thyroid health.
- **Anti-inflammatory Effects**: By reducing systemic inflammation, Ashwagandha may help manage thyroid dysfunction associated with autoimmune conditions like Hashimoto's thyroiditis or Graves' disease.

DOSAGE AND PRECAUTIONS

- **Typical Dosage**: 300–600 mg of standardized Ashwagandha extract daily is commonly recommended, but consultation with a healthcare provider is essential.
- **Precautions**: Not recommended for individuals with hyperthyroidism unless guided by a healthcare professional. Potential interactions with thyroid medications or other supplements.

BACOPA

Bramhi, scientifically known as *Bacopa Monnieri*, is a traditional Ayurvedic herb & serves as a nerve tonic and neuroprotective agent with a history of use in Ayurvedic medicine. Its long-standing reputation as a cognitive enhancer are well-known. Recent animal studies have demonstrated that Bacopa has the ability to boost thyroid function. One study found that an alcoholic extract of Bacopa can prevent hypothyroidism by increasing thyroid hormone production, improving antioxidant levels, lowering lipid profiles, and maintaining thyroid morphology. Another study looked at how Bacopa can protect against changes in thyroid hormone activity and its connection to Alzheimer's disease in rats. The research found that Bacopa significantly altered levels of T3 and T4 and indicators of neurodegeneration.

Brahmi is an adaptogenic herb known for its cognitive-enhancing and antioxidant properties. Research suggests it may impact thyroid health, especially in hypothyroidism, by potentially stimulating thyroid hormone production.

Here's a detailed summary of Bacopa monnieri’s potential effects on thyroid health:

IMPACT ON HYPOTHYROIDISM

- *Bacopa monnieri* may stimulate the thyroid gland to produce more T4 hormones.
- It may be a supportive therapy for hypothyroid patients.
- Neuroprotective properties of *Bacopa monnieri* may help alleviate cognitive deficits caused by hypothyroidism.

IMPACT ON HYPERTHYROIDISM

- Use with caution, as Bacopa monnieri might increase thyroid hormone levels.

- Not typically recommended for hyperthyroid conditions unless closely monitored by a healthcare provider.
- Overuse may risk overstimulation of the thyroid gland in individuals with normal or hyperthyroid conditions.

MECHANISM OF ACTION

- Bacopa monnieri may increase T4 levels (based on animal studies).
- Effects on T3 are less consistent.
- Rich in antioxidants, which help neutralize reactive oxygen species (ROS), protecting thyroid cells from damage and improving overall gland function.
- Anti-inflammatory properties may contribute to better thyroid health by reducing inflammation in the glandular tissues.

OTHER HEALTH BENEFITS

- **Stress Reduction**: Adaptogenic properties help reduce cortisol levels, indirectly supporting thyroid function as chronic stress negatively impacts thyroid health.
- **Cognitive Support**: May help alleviate cognitive dysfunction common in hypothyroidism.

SAFETY AND SIDE EFFECTS:

- **Interactions with Thyroid Medications**: May interact with synthetic thyroid hormones or antithyroid drugs, potentially altering their effectiveness.
- **Potential Overstimulation**: Overuse might risk overstimulation of the thyroid gland in individuals with normal or hyperthyroid conditions.
- Limited evidence on safety during pregnancy and breastfeeding.

Bacopa monnieri shows potential for supporting thyroid function, especially in hypothyroidism. However, more research, especially in humans, is needed to confirm its benefits. While it may support thyroid function by stimulating hormone production, individuals with thyroid disease, especially hyperthyroidism, should consult a doctor before use. Using Bacopa monnieri cautiously, especially alongside thyroid medications, is essential to avoid potential interactions.

NIGELLA SATIVA

Seeds of *Nigella Sativa*, commonly known as black cumin seeds, possess important health benefits including antioxidant, anti-inflammatory, and immune-boosting properties. Several animal studies have demonstrated the therapeutic advantages in various chronic illnesses such as diabetes, hyperlipidaemia, and hypertension; nevertheless, the protective function in hypothyroidism and particularly

Hashimoto's thyroiditis has been newly detected. The primary component in black cumin, which possesses antioxidant and anti-inflammatory characteristics, is **thymoquinone** and has also proven to enhance thyroid well-being in animal trials.

In a particular study, black cumin heightened T3 levels with no alteration in serum TSH levels. The ability of the substance to repair the thyroid gland, synthesize thyroid hormone, and enhance antioxidant defence systems contributes to its therapeutic effectiveness in reducing oxidative stress and protecting thyroid cells from damage and hyperplastic changes associated with thyroiditis.

EFFECTS ON HYPOTHYROIDISM

Nigella sativa (black seed) and its active compound, thymoquinone, have shown potential benefits for thyroid health, particularly in hypothyroidism. Research suggests that Nigella sativa may improve thyroid function by:

- **Increasing thyroid hormone levels:** Animal studies indicate that Nigella sativa may increase T3 and T4 hormone levels, possibly by enhancing thyroid peroxidase activity or reducing oxidative stress that can impair thyroid function.
- **Reducing inflammation**: Chronic inflammation can damage the thyroid gland. Nigella sativa's anti-inflammatory properties may

help reduce inflammation in the thyroid and surrounding tissues, potentially preventing tissue damage.

- **Modulating the immune system:** In autoimmune thyroid diseases like Hashimoto's thyroiditis and Graves' disease, the body's immune system attacks the thyroid gland. Nigella sativa's immunomodulatory effects may help regulate the immune system, reducing autoimmune attacks on the thyroid.
- **Improving metabolic disturbances:** Thyroid dysfunction, especially hypothyroidism, often leads to changes in cholesterol levels and metabolism. Nigella sativa's influence on lipid metabolism may help improve these metabolic disturbances.
- **Potential anti-cancer properties:** Preliminary research suggests that thymoquinone may inhibit the growth and proliferation of thyroid cancer cells. However, more clinical evidence is needed to support this claim.
- **Improved thyroid hormone levels in human studies:** Limited human clinical trials suggest that Nigella sativa may improve thyroid hormone levels in individuals with hypothyroidism.
- More research, particularly human clinical trials, is needed to fully understand Nigella sativa's role in thyroid health and its long-term effects. Individuals with thyroid conditions or on thyroid medication should consult a healthcare provider before using

Nigella sativa to determine the appropriate dosage and avoid potential interactions with medications.

TURMERIC

Turmeric, also known as *Curcuma longa*, is a plant species widely used for its health benefits. Turmeric, a common spice in culinary practices, has the ability to aid thyroid health through its strong anti-inflammatory characteristics. Curcumin, a bioactive compound present in turmeric, has been found to decrease thyroid inflammation and oxidative stress. Research on animals with induced hypothyroidism suggests that both turmeric and curcumin can boost thyroid function.

Curcuma longa (turmeric) and its active compound, curcumin, have been studied for their potential benefits on thyroid health. While more research is needed, here's a point-wise summary of the potential effects:

THYROID HORMONE REGULATION

- Some studies indicate that curcumin may increase T3 and T4 hormone levels in cases of hypothyroidism.
- Curcumin may also influence the conversion of T4 (inactive) to T3 (active), which may benefit those with hypothyroidism.
- There's some evidence that curcumin may reduce TSH levels, which is beneficial for people with hypothyroidism who often have high TSH levels.

ANTIOXIDANT EFFECTS

- Curcumin, a strong antioxidant, protects the thyroid gland from oxidative stress, which is linked to thyroid dysfunction.
- The thyroid gland is highly susceptible to oxidative damage due to its role in hormone production. Curcumin's antioxidant action may protect the gland and reduce the risk of dysfunction.
- Curcumin may also benefit individuals with both diabetes and thyroid disease, improving overall thyroid function by reducing insulin resistance and regulating glucose metabolism.

IMPACT ON AUTOIMMUNE THYROID CONDITIONS

- Curcumin may modulate the immune system and reduce inflammation in autoimmune disorders like Hashimoto's thyroiditis and Graves' disease.
- Curcumin has shown potential to reduce thyroid autoimmunity, particularly in Hashimoto's thyroiditis, where the immune system attacks the thyroid.

ANTI-CANCER EFFECTS

- In vitro studies show that curcumin inhibits the growth of thyroid cancer cells and may promote apoptosis (cell death) of malignant cells.
- Curcumin's anti-cancer effects are achieved through various pathways, including regulating inflammatory cytokines,

suppressing cell proliferation, and inhibiting tumor angiogenesis.

DOSAGE AND BIOAVAILABILITY

- Curcumin has poor bioavailability, meaning a small amount reaches the bloodstream. Combining it with piperine (found in black pepper) can increase its absorption.
- The optimal dosage of curcumin for thyroid health is not well-established, but general recommendations for supplements range from 500 to 2,000 mg per day. Starting with a lower dose and gradually increasing it is recommended, and consulting a healthcare provider is essential.

Curcuma longa (turmeric) and curcumin may offer benefits for thyroid health, particularly due to their anti-inflammatory, antioxidant, and immune-modulating properties. More research is needed to fully understand its therapeutic potential. Consult a healthcare provider before incorporating curcumin, especially for those with thyroid disorders or on medication.

Curcumin could interact with thyroid medications like levothyroxine, potentially affecting their effectiveness. It's crucial to consult a healthcare provider before taking curcumin if you are on thyroid medication.

GUGGUL

Obtained from the resin of the *Commiphora Mukul* tree, Guggul is an Ayurvedic plant commonly employed for treating diverse health issues like hypothyroidism. It is believed to have a positive impact on thyroid health through various mechanisms. It is believed that **guggulsterones**, the active ingredients in guggul, boost thyroid function by increasing the synthesis of thyroid hormones T_3 and T_4.

It has been demonstrated to possess antioxidant properties which can safeguard the thyroid gland against oxidative stress. While some research indicates potential benefits for thyroid function, more studies are required to confirm its efficacy and establish the best dosage.

Commiphora mukul, also known as Guggul, is a resin from the guggul tree used in Ayurvedic medicine. It may impact thyroid health, especially hypothyroidism, by possibly stimulating thyroid hormone production and regulating cholesterol levels. However, more research is needed to understand its exact mechanisms and effects on hyperthyroidism. Here's a detailed summary of Guggul's potential effects on thyroid health:

IMPACT ON HYPOTHYROIDISM:

- Guggul may stimulate the thyroid gland to produce more T3 and T4 hormones. Guggulsterones, compounds in Guggul, may regulate thyroid function.

- Guggul has lipid-lowering properties, which can benefit individuals with hypothyroidism who often have high cholesterol.
- Some studies suggest Guggul may influence thyroid function, but evidence is inconclusive, requiring more clinical studies in humans.

MECHANISM OF ACTION

- Guggulsterones may interact with thyroid receptors, influence thyroid metabolic processes, and regulate enzyme activity for better hormone production and secretion.
- Guggul may enhance iodine absorption in the thyroid gland, potentially supporting T3 and T4 production in hypothyroidism.
- Guggul's anti-inflammatory and antioxidant properties can improve overall thyroid health and protect the gland.

OTHER HEALTH BENEFITS

- **Weight Loss and Metabolism**: Guggul, traditionally used for weight management, may stimulate metabolism and aid in weight loss, especially in hypothyroid patients who experience weight gain.
- **Improved Cholesterol and Lipid Profile**: Guggul's lipid-lowering effects may regulate cholesterol, potentially improving cardiovascular health in those with thyroid dysfunction, especially

hypothyroidism, which often leads to elevated cholesterol levels.

- **Anti-Inflammatory Effects**: Guggul's anti-inflammatory properties can reduce systemic inflammation, which might benefit thyroid conditions like Hashimoto's thyroiditis or Graves' disease, although further research is needed.

SAFETY AND SIDE EFFECTS

- **Interactions with Thyroid Medications**: Guggul might interact with thyroid medications like levothyroxine, potentially causing hormonal imbalances.
- **Gastrointestinal Issues**: Some individuals may experience mild gastrointestinal discomfort, like diarrhea or nausea.
- **Hormonal Imbalance**: Overuse or misuse of Guggul might lead to hormonal imbalances if thyroid levels are not properly monitored.
- **Pregnancy and Breastfeeding**: Guggul should be avoided during pregnancy and breastfeeding due to limited research on its safety unless recommended by a healthcare provider.

Commiphora mukul (Guggul) shows promising effects on thyroid health, particularly in managing hypothyroidism symptoms and potentially balancing thyroid hormone levels. However, further research is necessary to confirm these benefits.

PUNARNAVA

Punarnava, also known as *Boerhavia diffusa*, is an Ayurvedic plant with a history of use in traditional medicine for many health issues and is thought to support thyroid function. Punarnava is recognized for its ability to increase urine production and reduce inflammation, which can impact the function of the thyroid. Certain studies indicate that Punarnava could potentially assist in controlling thyroid hormone levels, particularly by influencing T_3 (triiodothyronine) and T_4 (thyroxine). Additionally, Punarnava's anti-inflammatory qualities have the potential to decrease inflammation of the thyroid gland, which is crucial in autoimmune thyroid conditions.

While research primarily comes from animal studies and small-scale human trials, Boerhavia diffusa shows potential in managing oxidative stress and modulating thyroid activity, particularly in hyperthyroidism.

Here is a detailed summary of the potential effects of Boerhavia diffusa on thyroid health:

THYROID MODULATORY EFFECTS

- Boerhavia diffusa has adaptogenic and anti-inflammatory properties that may indirectly influence thyroid function.

- Some studies suggest that its extract can impact thyroid hormone levels (T3, T4, and TSH) by enhancing or suppressing production based on the physiological state.

ANTI-HYPERTHYROID ACTIVITY

- Boerhavia diffusa may have antithyroid activity, especially in cases of hyperthyroidism. Its bioactive components, including flavonoids and alkaloids, could suppress excessive thyroid activity by inhibiting thyroid peroxidase.

ANTIOXIDANT EFFECTS

- Boerhavia diffusa's potent antioxidant properties can protect thyroid tissue from oxidative damage, a factor linked to thyroid dysfunction.
- By reducing free radical production, it can help maintain thyroid health.

HEPATOPROTECTIVE ROLE

- Boerhavia diffusa has hepatoprotective effects that may support thyroid hormone metabolism.
- The liver is critical in this process, and improved liver function can aid in the proper metabolism and conversion of thyroid hormones.

TRADITIONAL AYURVEDIC PERSPECTIVE

- In **Ayurveda**, *Punarnava* is used to reduce swelling associated with thyroid diseases, particularly in hypothyroidism where edema is a common symptom.
- **Clinical Study**: One study evaluated the efficacy of a treatment containing Punarnavadi Kashaya, which includes Boerhavia diffusa. The study showed significant improvement in hypothyroidism symptoms, suggesting a supportive role for Boerhavia diffusa in thyroid health.

It's important to note that while Boerhavia diffusa has shown potential benefits, excessive or improper use could disrupt thyroid function or interact with thyroid medications. Individuals considering its use should consult healthcare professionals.

-$$$-

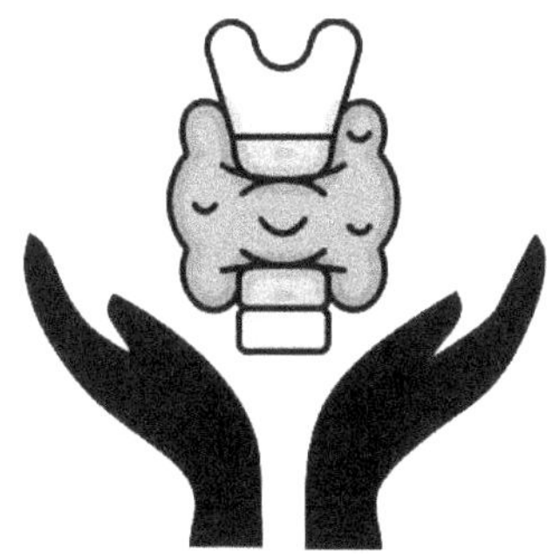

Nutrients for Healthy Thyroid

Dr Surabhi Singh

This chapter explores the essential nutrients that play crucial roles in maintaining optimal thyroid health. The thyroid gland, responsible for producing hormones that regulate metabolism, growth, and energy production, relies on a delicate balance of these nutrients. Deficiencies in any of these can lead to thyroid dysfunction and impact overall well-being. Numerous nutrients are important for maintaining thyroid health. Furthermore, individuals with hypothyroidism have a higher likelihood of lacking specific nutrients compared to others.

IODINE: THE CORNERSTONE OF THYROID HORMONE

A lack of iodine can lead to hypothyroidism because this mineral is essential for creating thyroid hormones. Insufficient consumption of iodine is actually the leading cause of hypothyroidism across the globe. While iodine deficiency is prevalent in some areas globally, it is not as widespread in developed nations. Those at higher risk of low iodine levels include individuals who do not consume iodized salt, pregnant women, and individuals following a vegan diet.

If you have hypothyroidism, do not take iodine supplements unless advised by a doctor to address low iodine levels. Excessive iodine intake can be detrimental to the thyroid and may cause hyperthyroidism in individuals residing in regions with high iodine content.

IMPORTANT FACTS

- Iodine is the most critical nutrient for thyroid function, as it is a fundamental component of the thyroid hormones T3 (triiodothyronine) and T4 (thyroxine).
- The thyroid gland actively concentrates iodine from the bloodstream via the sodium-iodide symporter (NIS) and utilizes it to synthesize thyroid hormones.
- Iodine deficiency leads to reduced T3 and T4 production, triggering a compensatory increase in thyroid-stimulating hormone (TSH) from the pituitary gland.
- Chronic iodine deficiency can cause goiter (enlarged thyroid) and hypothyroidism. Severe deficiency during fetal development can lead to cretinism, characterized by stunted growth and cognitive impairments.

- The recommended daily intake (RDA) of iodine is 150 µg/day for adults, with increased requirements during pregnancy (220 µg/day) and lactation (290 µg/day).
- Good sources of iodine include iodized salt, seafood, dairy products, and certain seaweeds.

SELENIUM: THE ANTIOXIDANT SHIELD AND HORMONE ACTIVATOR

Selenium is vital for the health of the thyroid gland and the synthesis of thyroid hormones. Incorporating selenium-rich foods into your diet is beneficial for safeguarding the thyroid gland against oxidative stress-induced harm and for boosting selenium levels. In addition, some individuals with hypothyroidism may find selenium supplements helpful. A study from 2023 indicates that taking 200 mcg of selenium daily can decrease thyroid antibodies and alleviate symptoms like low mood in those with Hashimoto's thyroiditis. Nevertheless, selenium supplements are not essential for all individuals with hypothyroidism.

IMPORTANT FACTS

- Selenium, a trace mineral, is crucial for thyroid hormone metabolism and antioxidant defence.
- Selenium is incorporated into **selenoproteins**, including deiodinase enzymes, which convert T4 to the active T3.
- Selenium also protects the thyroid gland from oxidative damage

by neutralizing reactive oxygen species (ROS) as part of thioredoxin reductase.

- Selenium deficiency impairs deiodinase function, reducing T3 levels and compromising thyroid hormone activation. This can lead to hypothyroidism, and in severe cases, Keshan disease (a cardiomyopathy).
- Selenium deficiency is also linked to an increased risk of autoimmune thyroid diseases like Hashimoto's thyroiditis.
- The RDA for selenium is 55 µg/day for adults. Individuals with autoimmune thyroid conditions may benefit from higher selenium levels to reduce inflammation and improve thyroid function.
- Consistent consumption of high levels of selenium can lead to hair and nail loss, diarrhoea, nausea, and rashes.
- Severe selenium poisoning can result in potentially life-threatening effects like kidney failure, heart attack, and breathing difficulties.
- Brazil nuts are the richest source of selenium, followed by seafood, meats, eggs, and whole grains.

ZINC: THE ORCHESTRATOR OF THYROID HORMONE SYNTHESIS AND SENSITIVITY

Zinc, similar to selenium, is essential for the production of thyroid hormones and overall thyroid health. A lack of zinc in your diet can impact thyroid function and lead to various health issues, emphasizing the importance of sufficient zinc intake. Zinc supplements can enhance thyroid function in hypothyroid patients when used alone or in conjunction with selenium and vitamin-A.

In addition to the nutrients mentioned before, there are other vitamins and minerals that should be taken into account for individuals with hypothyroidism.

IMPORTANT FACTS

- Zinc is vital for the synthesis, activation, and regulation of thyroid hormones.
- It acts as a co-factor in various enzymatic processes, including thyroid hormone synthesis and TSH secretion.
- Zinc also enhances the action of thyroid hormone receptors, ensuring proper cellular responses to T3.
- Zinc deficiency can reduce thyroid hormone production and impair the response to thyroid hormones, leading to hypothyroidism and metabolic slowing.
- Zinc deficiency may also contribute to autoimmune thyroid diseases by impairing the immune system.
- The RDA for zinc is 11 mg/day for men and 8 mg/day for women. Vegetarians may need supplementation due to the lower bioavailability of zinc from plant-based sources.

- Good sources of zinc include red meat, shellfish, legumes, seeds, and nuts.

VITAMIN D: THE IMMUNE MODULATOR FOR THYROID HEALTH

Individuals who have hypothyroidism have a higher tendency to lack essential nutrients. Inadequate levels of vitamin D can impact thyroid function and exacerbate hypothyroidism symptoms. Due to the lack of high levels of vitamin D in a variety of foods, taking supplements is frequently needed.

IMPORTANT FACTS

- Vitamin D plays an indirect but significant role in thyroid health through immune modulation.
- Its active form, 1,25-dihydroxyvitamin D, binds to vitamin D receptors in the thyroid gland, influencing thyroid hormone production and immune cell differentiation.
- Vitamin D's anti-inflammatory properties can prevent autoimmune thyroid diseases by modulating cytokine production and T-cell activity.
- Low vitamin D levels are linked to an increased risk of autoimmune thyroid diseases, especially Hashimoto's thyroiditis. Deficiency may worsen thyroid dysfunction and impair immune regulation of thyroid function.
- The RDA for vitamin D is 600-800 IU/day for adults, with higher

requirements during pregnancy and in older adults. Some studies suggest higher doses may be beneficial for thyroid function and immune regulation.

- Vitamin D is primarily obtained through sun exposure, and it is also found in fatty fish, fortified dairy products, and egg yolks.

VITAMIN B12: THE METABOLIC AND NEUROLOGICAL SUPPORT

Hypothyroid patients frequently experience a lack of Vitamin B12. Vit. B12 deficiency can mimic or worsen hypothyroidism symptoms, such as fatigue and cognitive impairment. Long-term deficiency can cause neurological damage, especially in individuals with thyroid dysfunction. Vitamin B12 is essential for red blood cell synthesis, neurological function, and energy production.

IMPORTANT POINTS

- It plays a role in methylation processes that influence gene expression related to thyroid health.
- Vitamin B12 is involved in converting homocysteine to methionine, indirectly affecting thyroid hormone metabolism.
- B12 deficiency is common in individuals with hypothyroidism, particularly those with autoimmune thyroid diseases.
- The RDA for vitamin B12 is 2.4 µg/day for adults. Higher amounts may be needed for those with gastrointestinal issues or strict vegetarian diets.

- Vitamin B12 is found in animal-based products like meat, fish, poultry, dairy, and eggs. Fortified foods or supplements may be necessary for those on a plant-based diet.

MAGNESIUM: THE FACILITATOR OF THYROID HORMONE ACTION

Low levels of magnesium are linked to hypothyroidism and can raise the likelihood of developing hypothyroidism. Supplementing with magnesium has been demonstrated to enhance hypothyroidism.

IMPORTANT FACTS

- Magnesium is involved in over 300 enzymatic processes, including those related to thyroid hormone synthesis and metabolism.
- It helps regulate the conversion of T4 to T3 and is essential for the Na+/K+-ATPase pump, which maintains the thyroid cell's electrical balance.
- Magnesium promotes thyroid hormone action by supporting enzymes involved in T4-to-T3 conversion, contributing to overall metabolic balance.
- It also reduces stress-related cortisol production, which can suppress thyroid function.
- Magnesium deficiency has been linked to lower T3 levels, increased cortisol, and reduced thyroid hormone receptor

sensitivity. This can lead to hypothyroidism symptoms and metabolic dysregulation.

- The RDA for magnesium is 400-420 mg/day for men and 310-320 mg/day for women, with higher needs during stress and illness.
- Magnesium-rich foods include leafy green vegetables, nuts, seeds, legumes, and whole grains.

TYROSINE: THE BUILDING BLOCK OF THYROID HORMONES

Tyrosine is a crucial amino acid that plays a vital role in thyroid function. Tyrosine supplementation should not be considered a replacement for conventional thyroid hormone replacement therapy (levothyroxine) prescribed by a healthcare professional. Here's a breakdown of its importance:

BUILDING BLOCK FOR THYROID HORMONES

Tyrosine serves as the foundation for the synthesis of thyroid hormones:

- **Thyroxine (T4):** This is the primary hormone produced by the thyroid gland.
- **Triiodothyronine (T3):** This is the more active form of thyroid hormone, converted from T4.

IMPORTANT FACTS

- The thyroid gland combines tyrosine with iodine to produce T4 and T3.
- Tyrosine, an amino acid, serves as a precursor to thyroid hormones T3 and T4.
- It combines with iodine to form thyroid hormones, making it particularly important for individuals with hypothyroidism.
- Tyrosine deficiency can reduce thyroid hormone production, leading to symptoms of low thyroid function.
- While the body can produce tyrosine from phenylalanine, supplementation is sometimes recommended for individuals with thyroid problems or high stress.
- Tyrosine is found in high-protein foods such as chicken, turkey, dairy, soy products, and legumes.

IRON: CO-FACTOR IN THYROID HORMONE SYNTHESIS

Iron is an essential mineral that plays a crucial role in various bodily functions, including thyroid hormone production and metabolism. Reduced iron levels or iron deficiency anaemia can impact thyroid function. Taking dietary supplements is frequently needed in order to reach and uphold optimal iron levels. Here's a breakdown of its importance in thyroid health:

THYROID HORMONE SYNTHESIS

- Iron is a cofactor for thyroid peroxidase (TPO), an enzyme that plays a critical role in thyroid hormone synthesis.
- TPO is responsible for:
    - **Iodide oxidation:** This is the process of converting iodide to iodine, which is necessary for thyroid hormone production.
    - **Iodination of thyroglobulin:** This is the process of attaching iodine to thyroglobulin, a protein that serves as the precursor for thyroid hormones.
- Inadequate iron levels can impair TPO activity, leading to decreased thyroid hormone production.

CONVERSION OF T4 TO T3

- T4 is the primary hormone produced by the thyroid gland, but T3 is the more active form that exerts most of the thyroid hormone effects on target tissues.
- The conversion of T4 to T3 occurs mainly in peripheral tissues, such as the liver and kidneys.
- Iron is involved in this conversion process, and iron deficiency may impair the conversion of T4 to T3, leading to reduced T3 levels.

THYROID HORMONE METABOLISM

- Iron is also involved in the metabolism of thyroid hormones, including their breakdown and clearance from the body.
- Iron deficiency may affect thyroid hormone metabolism, potentially leading to imbalances in thyroid hormone levels.

IRON DEFICIENCY AND HYPOTHYROIDISM

- Iron deficiency is often associated with hypothyroidism, particularly in women of reproductive age.
- Iron deficiency can exacerbate the symptoms of hypothyroidism, such as fatigue, weakness, and cold intolerance.
- Correcting iron deficiency may improve thyroid function and reduce hypothyroid symptoms.

-$$$-

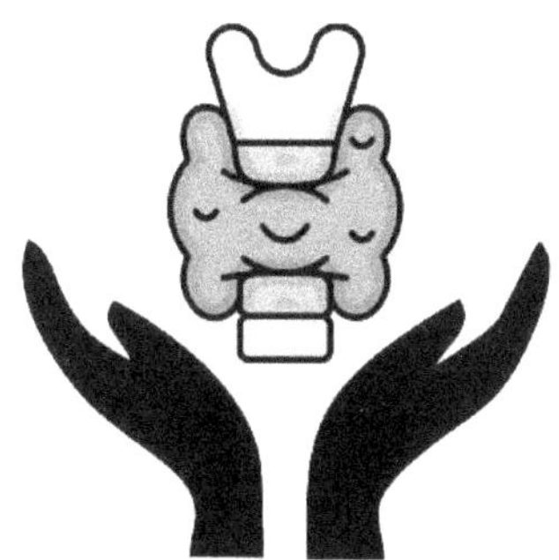

Foods For Healthy Thyroid

Dr Muskan Maurya

Eating a balanced diet will keep the thyroid healthy. You don't have to eliminate a lot of foods, but certain foods may be problematic for individuals with hypothyroidism. There may be a lot of claims regarding diets for hypothyroidism. However, there is no proof that eating or avoiding particular foods can improve thyroid function in those who have an underactive thyroid.

WHY DIET MATTERS FOR THYROID HEALTH

1. Supports Thyroid Hormone Production- Essential nutrients like iodine, selenium, and zinc are required for the synthesis and activation of thyroid hormones.

2. Reduces Inflammation- Anti-inflammatory foods can help manage autoimmune thyroid conditions like Hashimoto's and Graves' disease.

3. Balances Weight -Thyroid conditions can affect metabolism, leading to weight gain or loss. A proper diet can help to regulate body weight.

4. Improves Energy Levels- Nutrient-rich foods help combat fatigue often associated with thyroid disorders.

5. Manages Symptoms- Certain foods can exacerbate or alleviate symptoms like brain fog, hair loss, or sensitivity to cold/heat.

FOODS THAT SHOULD BE AVOIDED

A thyroid-friendly diet plays a crucial role in supporting thyroid health and managing conditions like hypothyroidism, hyperthyroidism, or Hashimoto's thyroiditis. The thyroid gland regulates metabolism, energy levels, and overall hormonal balance.

GLUTEN AND HIGHLY PROCESSED FOODS

Gluten is a type of protein present in wheat, barley, and rye. Some studies propose that individuals with Hashimoto's thyroiditis could see advantages from adopting a diet free of gluten. Different studies from credible sources have conflicting views on the necessity of a gluten-free diet for all individuals.

In addition, individuals with hypothyroidism should consider restricting certain foods to improve their overall well-being. For instance, those with Hashimoto's thyroiditis exhibit elevated levels of inflammation and oxidative stress. Oxidative stress is defined by an abundance of reactive molecules in the body known as free radicals, which overpower the body's anti-oxidant defences and can lead to cell harm.

Those with hypothyroidism should steer clear of foods that trigger oxidative stress and inflammation, like processed foods, sugary foods and drinks, and fried foods. Along with oxidative stress, a diet rich in these foods is associated with obesity, so cutting back on their consumption can assist individuals in maintaining a healthy weight.

GOITROGENS

Substances like goitrogens are present in cruciferous vegetables like cabbage and Brussels sprouts, as well as soy products, and can block the production of thyroid hormone. The majority of individuals, even those with hypothyroidism, can consume moderate quantities of goiter-inducing foods without negatively impacting their thyroid health.

Cruciferous vegetables such as broccoli have a high content of goitre. Furthermore, cooking these foods decreases their goitrogenic activity, which is beneficial for individuals with hypothyroidism. Nevertheless, it is advisable to refrain from juicing extensive quantities of raw cruciferous vegetables.

FOODS THAT CAN BE EATEN

Consuming a diet full of healthy, nutrient-dense foods can enhance overall well-being and support weight management. Furthermore, elevated levels of this nutrient could potentially decrease the likelihood of developing health issues linked to hypothyroidism like heart disease, obesity, and type 2 diabetes. A high-fiber diet can also help reduce the risk of constipation, a common symptom of hypothyroidism. If you have hypothyroidism, try adding the following nutritious foods to your diet:

- **Starchy vegetables**: greens, artichokes, squash, asparagus, carrots, peppers, spinach or mushrooms
- **Fruits**: berries, apples, peaches, pears, grapes, citrus fruits, pineapple or bananas
- **Fish, eggs, meat and poultry**: fish and shellfish, eggs, turkey or chicken
- **Healthy fats**: olive oil, avocados, avocado oil, coconut oil, unsweetened coconut, or full-fat yogurt
- **Gluten-free grains**: brown rice, oats, quinoa, or brown rice pasta
- **Seeds, nuts, and nut butters**: almonds, cashews, macadamia nuts, walnuts, pumpkin seeds, or natural peanut butter
- **Beans and lentils**: chickpeas, beans or lentils
- **Milk and milk substitutes**: coconut milk, cashew milk, coconut yogurt, almond milk, unsweetened yogurt or cheese,
- **Herbs & Spices**: spices such as paprika, saffron or turmeric, fresh or dried herbs like basil or rosemary, and spices like salsa or mustard.

- **Beverages**: water, unsweetened tea, coffee or mineral water

Keep in mind that certain individuals with an underactive thyroid might see positive results from eliminating gluten and dairy from their diet. Other individuals may not have to remove these foods from their eating habits and can ingest gluten and dairy without any issues.

It is crucial to develop a personalized nutrition plan that fits your individual health requirements. If possible, collaborate with a certified dietitian to identify which foods you should remove from your diet. They can also assist you in creating a well-rounded meal plan that includes all essential nutrients without excluding any nutritious ingredients.

-$$$-

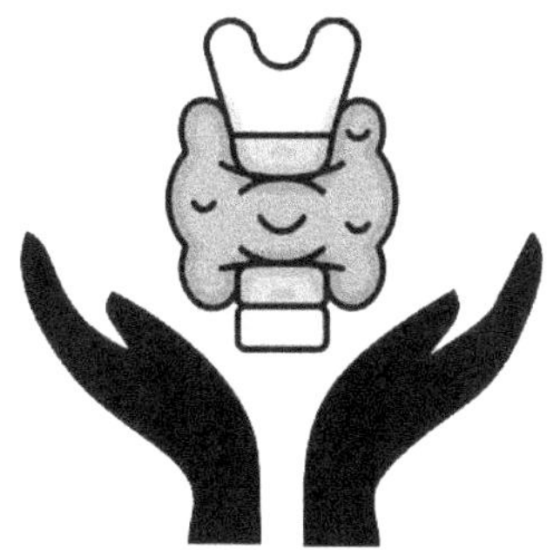

Yoga For Hypothyroidism

Dr. Abdul Vahid

Yoga can be a beneficial complementary therapy for managing hypothyroidism. Certain yoga poses are thought to stimulate the thyroid gland and improve circulation in the throat area, which may help in balancing thyroid function. Here are some yoga practices and poses that are often recommended.

Ujjayi Pranayama: Also known as the "*Victorious Breath*," this breathing technique involves a slight constriction of the throat and can help to stimulate the thyroid gland.

Sarvangasana: The "Shoulder Stand" is believed to improve the efficiency of the thyroid by increasing blood flow to the gland.

Halasana: Known as the "Plow Pose," this asana stretches the neck and stimulates the thyroid.

Setu Bandhasana: The "Bridge Pose" is another posture that can potentially benefit thyroid function.

Bhujangasana: The "Cobra Pose" helps to open up the chest and regulate the thyroid.

It's important to practice these poses under the guidance of a qualified yoga instructor, especially if you are new to yoga or have any health concerns. Additionally, always consult with your healthcare provider before starting any new exercise regimen to ensure it's appropriate for your condition.

For a more structured practice, you might consider following a yoga routine specifically designed for thyroid health, such as the ones available in online tutorials. These routines often include a combination of asanas, pranayama, and meditation to address the symptoms of hypothyroidism holistically. Remember, while yoga can support thyroid health, it should not replace any medical treatments prescribed by your doctor. It's best used as a complementary approach alongside your existing treatment plan.

UJJAYI PRANAYAMA

Ujjayi Pranayama, often referred to as the "*Victorious Breath*," is a key component of yoga practice that can be particularly beneficial for thyroid health. Here's a step-by-step guide to practicing Ujjayi Pranayama:

STEPS

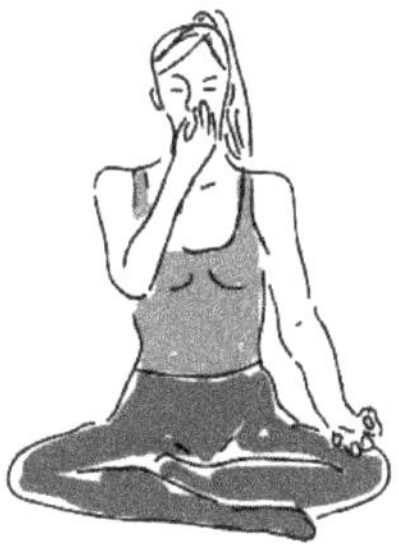

- **Find a Comfortable Seat**: Sit in a stable and comfortable position, such as *Sukhasana* (Easy Pose), with your spine erect.
- **Close Your Mouth**: Keep your mouth closed throughout the practice.
- **Constrict the Throat**: Gently constrict the back of your throat, the glottis, which is the part of the larynx around the vocal cords.
- **Inhale Slowly**: Begin to inhale slowly and deeply through your nose, allowing the air to create a friction sound as it passes through the constricted throat.
- **Sense of Fullness**: Continue inhaling until you feel a sense of fullness in your chest.
- **Retention**: If comfortable and advised by a teacher, retain the breath for about 6 seconds, or double the duration of your inhalation.
- **Relax the Face**: Ensure that your facial muscles are relaxed and that there's no constriction in the nostrils.
- **Exhale Naturally**: Exhale slowly and naturally, allowing the breath to leave your body without force.
- **Repeat**: Practice several rounds of Ujjayi breathing, maintaining a smooth and rhythmic pattern.

RECOMMENDED PRACTICE

Start with 5 rounds of Ujjayi breathing, gradually increasing the duration as per your comfort. It's important to practice without strain and to avoid retention of breath if you have cardiac or hypertension issues.

BENEFITS

Ujjayi Pranayama is known to help clear phlegm, increase appetite, and stimulate and balance the thyroid, among other benefits. Remember to practice Ujjayi Pranayama under the guidance of a qualified instructor, especially if you're new to it or have any health concerns.

HALASANA

Halasana, or the Plow Pose, is a yoga asana that offers several benefits, including stimulation of the thyroid gland. Here's how to perform *Halasana*.

STEPS

- **Starting Position**: Lie on your back with your arms beside you, palms facing down.
- **Inhale and Lift**: As you inhale, use your abdominal muscles to lift your feet off the floor, raising your legs vertically at a 90-degree angle.

- **Support Your Hips**: Continue to breathe normally and, supporting your hips and back with your hands, lift them off the ground.
- **Legs Overhead**: Allow your legs to sweep in a 180-degree angle over your head until your toes touch the floor. Your back should be perpendicular to the floor. This may be difficult initially, but make an attempt for a few seconds.

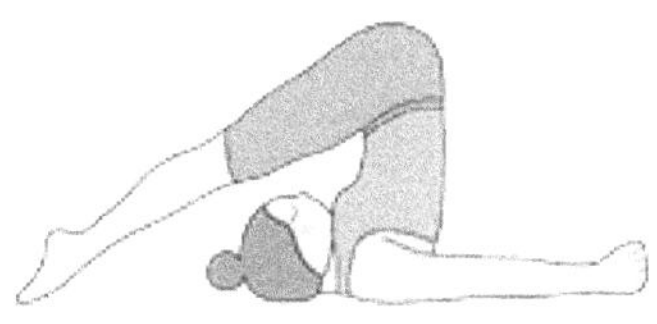

- **Hold the Pose**: Hold this pose and let your body relax more and more with each steady breath. For beginners, a few seconds are sufficient. Gradually, you can increase the duration.
- **Release**: After about a minute (or a comfortable duration for you), you may gently bring your legs down on exhalation.

TIPS FOR HALASANA

- Perform *Halasana* slowly and gently to avoid straining your neck or pushing it into the ground1.
- Ensure that you do not jerk your body while bringing the legs down.
- If you have any health concerns, such as neck injury, high blood pressure, or if you are pregnant, it's best to avoid this pose or consult a doctor before practicing.

- Remember to practice yoga within your own limits and comfort levels, and it's always recommended to learn new poses under the guidance of a qualified yoga instructor.

SARVANGASANA

Sarvangasana, also known as the Shoulder Stand, is a beneficial yoga pose for overall well-being, including thyroid health. Here's a step-by-step guide to performing *Sarvangasana*.

STEPS FOR SARVANGASANA

- **Preparation**: Begin by lying flat on your back with your arms by your side, palms facing down.
- **Lift**: Inhale and lift your legs, buttocks, and back in one smooth motion so that you come up high on your shoulders.
- **Support**: Place your hands on your back for support, moving your elbows closer towards each other and creeping your hands up towards your shoulder blades.
- **Align**: Straighten your legs and spine by pressing your elbows down into the floor and your hands into your back, ensuring your weight is supported on your shoulders and upper arms, not on your head and neck.

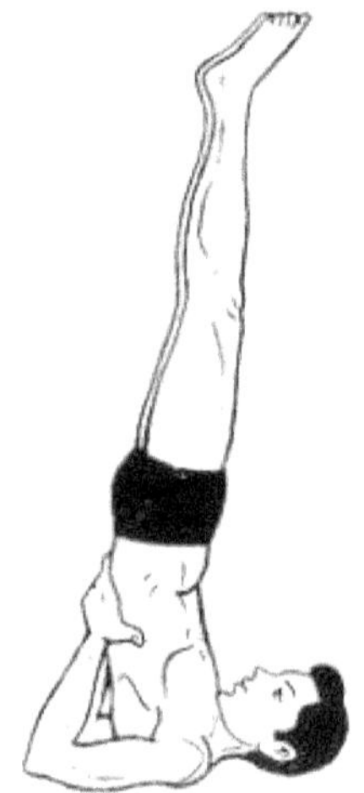

- **Position of Legs**: Lift your heels higher as if you are putting a footprint on the ceiling. Bring your big toes straight over your nose, then point the toes upwards.

- **Neck Position**: Be mindful of your neck. Do not press it into the floor; instead, keep it strong with a slight tightening of the neck muscles.
- **Hold**: Breathe deeply and hold the posture for 30-60 seconds, depending on your comfort level.
- **Exit**: To exit the pose, lower your knees to your forehead, place your hands on the floor with palms down, and slowly roll your spine down, vertebra by vertebra, to the floor. Lower your legs to the floor and relax.

IMPORTANT NOTE

If you have any health conditions like high blood pressure, heart problems, or neck pain, consult your physician before attempting *Sarvangasana*. It's also recommended to practice this pose under the guidance of a qualified yoga instructor. Remember, the key to a successful practice is to perform each step mindfully and without rushing, respecting your body's limits.

BHUJANGASANA

Bhujangasana, or Cobra Pose, is a rejuvenating backbend that strengthens the spine and can be therapeutic for the thyroid. Here's how to perform it:

STEPS FOR BHUJANGASANA

- **Start Position**: Lie flat on your stomach with your toes flat on the floor, and your forehead resting on the ground.
- **Hand Placement**: Place your hands under your shoulders with palms down and elbows close to your body.
- **Inhale and Lift**: Taking a deep breath in, slowly lift your head, chest, and abdomen while keeping your navel on the floor.
- **Support with Hands**: Use your hands to pull your torso back and off the floor, distributing the bend evenly across your spine.
- **Elbows Bent**: Keep your elbows slightly bent and shoulders away from your ears.
- **Gaze Up**: If comfortable, tilt your head back and look up, deepening the stretch in your chest and neck.
- **Hold the Pose**: Maintain the pose for 4-5 breaths, ensuring even breathing.
- **Exhale and Lower**: Breathe out and gently bring your abdomen, chest, and head back to the floor.
- **Relax**: Relax on the floor before repeating the pose if desired.

TIPS FOR BEGINNERS

- Keep the feet together or hip-width apart, depending on your comfort.
- Engage your thighs and firm your buttocks to support the lower back.
- Start with a gentle arch and gradually increase the depth as your flexibility improves.
- Avoid straining your back; the lift should come from the strength of your back muscles rather than pushing with your hands.

If you have any back issues, consult with a healthcare provider before attempting this pose. It's always best to learn yoga poses under the guidance of a qualified instructor.

Remember, the goal of *Bhujangasana* is not to achieve the deepest backbend but to find a balance between strength and flexibility, creating a sensation of lengthening and opening in the spine.

- $$$

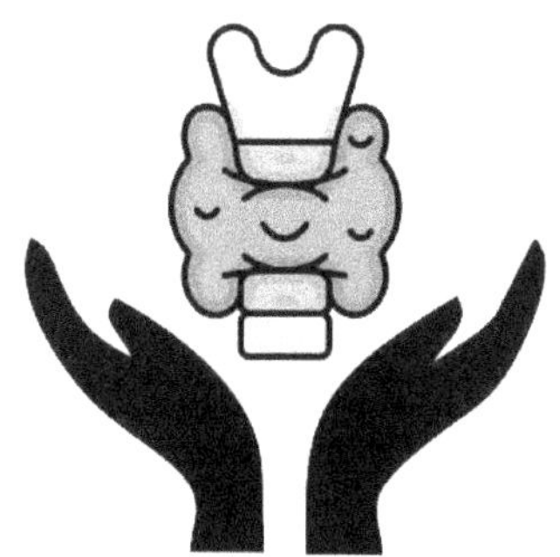

Research & Case Studies

Dr. Ajay Kumar, Dr. Abhishek Yadav, Dr. Abdul Vahid

Various research studies suggests that **Ayurveda** views hypothyroidism as a manifestation of deeper imbalances within the body, rather than just a deficiency of thyroid hormones. Several key concepts emerge:

- **Agni** (**Digestive Fire**): In **Ayurveda**, *Agni* represents the body's metabolic fire responsible for digestion and transformation at all levels. Sources emphasize the role of *Agni* in maintaining overall health and its disruption in hypothyroidism. Specifically, the concept of *Agnimandya* (low digestive fire) is associated with hypothyroidism, leading to impaired metabolism and various symptoms.
- **Ama** (**Toxins**): *Ama* is undigested metabolic waste that can accumulate in the body and disrupt various physiological

processes. *Ama* is implicated in the development of various diseases, including autoimmune conditions like hypothyroidism. This accumulation can further hinder *Agni* and exacerbate the existing imbalances.

- **Dosha Imbalances**: **Ayurveda** recognizes three fundamental energies or *Doshas* – *Vata, Pitta*, and *Kapha* – that govern various bodily functions. Imbalances in these *Doshas* are believed to be the root cause of diseases. While the specific *Dosha* imbalances can vary among individuals with hypothyroidism, *Kapha* imbalances, characterized by slow metabolism, fluid retention, and weight gain, are often implicated. *Kapha* and *Meda* (fat) are main contributing factors in the formation of nodules, and *Agnimandya* is linked at the systemic and cellular level with hypothyroidism.

AYURVEDIC TREATMENT PRINCIPLES

Ayurveda's approach to managing hypothyroidism involves restoring balance to *Agni*, eliminating *Ama*, and correcting *Dosha* imbalances through various therapeutic strategies:

- **Shodhana (Purification)**: Purification therapies aim to eliminate accumulated toxins (*Ama*) and restore the body's natural balance. These therapies often involve *Panchakarma* procedures like *Vamana* (therapeutic vomiting), *Virechana* (purgation), and *Basti* (therapeutic enemas), as exemplified in studies.

- **Shamana (Palliative)**: Palliative therapies focus on alleviating symptoms and supporting the body's healing process. This typically involves herbal formulations tailored to the individual's specific *Dosha* imbalances and presenting symptoms. Examples of such formulations mentioned in the sources include *Yashtimadhu, Dhatri Loha, Nityananda Rasa, Vyoshadi Guggulu*, and *Shadushana Churna*.
- **Dietary and Lifestyle Modifications**: **Ayurveda** strongly emphasizes the role of diet and lifestyle in maintaining health and managing diseases. Specific dietary recommendations for hypothyroidism often involve avoiding heavy, difficult-to-digest foods that can contribute to *Ama* formation, while favouring warm, cooked foods that support *Agni*. Lifestyle modifications may include regular exercise, stress management techniques, and adequate sleep.

CASE STUDY - 1

This study discusses an Ayurvedic approach to treating hypothyroidism. They describe a case study of a 27-year-old woman who presented with symptoms of both rheumatoid arthritis (RA) and subclinical hypothyroidism.

In **Ayurveda**, hypothyroidism is believed to be caused by an imbalance of the three *Doshas*: *Vata*, *Pitta*, and *Kapha*. Specifically, hypothyroidism is seen as a *Santarpanottha* (over nourishment) condition of *Kapha Meda* origin. *Ama*, which is a toxic byproduct of undigested food, is also believed to play a role in the development of hypothyroidism. The authors argue that hypothyroidism and RA, both of which are autoimmune diseases, share a similar pathogenesis related to *Ama*.

In this case study, the patient was treated with a variety of Ayurvedic therapies, including *Koshtha Shuddhi, Deepana* and *Pachana*, followed by *Kshara Basti*. The authors explain that these therapies were chosen because they target *Ama*, improve *Agni*, and ultimately address the root cause of the disease.

KOSHTHA SHUDDHI

- *Koshtha Shuddhi* is a mild Ayurvedic purgation therapy that is used to cleanse the digestive tract and improve digestion. It involves the oral administration of *Gandharvahastadi-Erandatailam*, *Shivakshara Pachana Churna*, and *Shunthi Siddha Jala*.
- In the case study, *Koshtha Shuddhi* was administered for five days before *Kshara Basti*. This was done to clear the patient's constipation, which is thought to contribute to hypothyroidism.

DEEPANA AND PACHANA

- *Deepana* and *Pachana* are Ayurvedic therapies that stimulate and promote digestion, respectively.
- The purpose of performing *Deepana* and *Pachana* prior to *Kshara Basti* was to ensure better absorption and bioavailability of the drugs used in the enema.
- *Shivakshara Pachana Churna*, which has *Teekshna* (penetrating) and *Ushna Guna* (hot properties), was used to neutralize *Ama* and clear *Srotovibandha* (obstruction of channels). This, in turn, helped to reduce the patient's pain and morning stiffness.

KSHARA BASTI

- *Kshara Basti* is an Ayurvedic therapeutic enema that is traditionally used to treat *Amavata*. The authors of the case study explain that they chose to use *Kshara Basti* to treat hypothyroidism because the pathogenesis of hypothyroidism is believed to be similar to that of *Amavata*.
- *Kshara Basti* is made up of several ingredients, including *Saindhava* (rock salt), *Guda* (jaggery), *Chincha* (tamarind), *Shatahva* (*Anethum sowa*), and *Gomutra* (cow's urine). These ingredients are believed to work together to neutralize *Ama*, clear *Samata* and *Srotorodha*, and reduce the symptoms of both RA

and hypothyroidism.

- *Kshara Basti* was administered daily for five days after the patient received *Koshtha Shuddhi*. To avoid weakness, the patient was advised to eat *Mudgayusha* (soup made of green gram) in the morning a few hours before each administration of the enema.

Following treatment with *Kshara Basti*, the patient experienced substantial relief in her symptoms. Her TSH levels decreased from 31.1 µIU/ml to 16.6 µIU/ml within 10 days. Her T_3 and T_4 levels also initially decreased, but then rose closer to normal levels after two months. The patient also experienced relief from her RA symptoms, including pain, stiffness, and deformity in her right little finger.

Case Study-1: Source: - Singh K, Rais A, Thakar AB. Management of hypothyroidism by Kshara Basti (therapeutic enema) A case report. AYU 2019; 40:237-41

CASE STUDY - 2

This is a case study from the *Journal of* ***Ayurveda*** *and Integrative Medical Sciences* that examines the Ayurvedic management of hypothyroidism. This case study reports on the treatment of a 38-year-old female patient who had been experiencing weight gain, fatigue, and hair loss for six months and had been diagnosed with hypothyroidism ten years prior. The study highlights the Ayurvedic perspective on hypothyroidism and the treatment approach used, focusing on the use of *Shamanoushadhi* (herbal medicines) and

Rasayana (rejuvenating therapies).

The case study begins by describing the patient's presentation and medical history. The patient was experiencing a range of symptoms commonly associated with hypothyroidism, including weight gain, fatigue, hair loss, indigestion, and dry skin. She had been on 75 mg of Thyroxine daily for the past ten years. The case study emphasizes that the clinical presentation of hypothyroidism often resembles *Sthoulya* (obesity) in **Ayurveda**, and therefore the treatment strategy should be aligned with *Sthoulya Chikitsa* (treatment for obesity).

The Ayurvedic treatment approach for this patient involved a combination of *Shodhana* (purification therapies), *Shamana* (palliative therapies), and *Vyadhihara Rasayana* (disease-specific rejuvenation therapies). The specific treatment plan for the patient included:

- **Yashtimadhu (licorice) capsules**: Two capsules were administered three times a day before meals with lukewarm water. *Yashtimadhu* is known for its beneficial effects on dry skin.
- **Dhatri Loha tablets**: One tablet was given three times a day before meals with lukewarm water. *Dhatri Loha* is believed to address indigestion and act as a *Rasayana*.
- **Nityananda Rasa tablets**: Two tablets were administered three times a day after meals with lukewarm water. *Nityananda Rasa*

is considered beneficial for *Mamsa Medogata Vikaras* (disorders affecting muscle and fat tissue). The authors explain that since *Sthoulya* is primarily a *Meda Pradhana Vyadhi* (disease dominated by fat imbalance), *Nityananda Rasa*, with its *Vata Kaphahara* (balancing *Vata* and *Kapha Doshas*), *Lekhana* (scraping), and *Rasayana* properties, was included in the treatment regimen.

- **Dietary Recommendations**: The patient was advised to follow a light diet and include barley (*Yava*) in her meals. Barley is known for its *Rukshana* (drying) property, which is thought to help reduce excess fat.
- **Exercise**: The patient was also encouraged to engage in exercises.

The case study reports that after two months of treatment, the patient experienced a significant reduction in her symptoms, with a 60% overall improvement. Her weight decreased from 73 kg to 70 kg. Additionally, her thyroid profile showed improvements, with TSH levels decreasing from 49.60 µIU/ml to 12.0 µIU/ml.

The authors conclude that the combination of Nityananda Rasa, *Yashtimadhu*, *Dhatri Loha*, dietary modifications, and exercise was effective in managing the patient's hypothyroidism. They acknowledge that the study's findings are based on a single case and suggest further research with larger patient groups to validate the results.

This case study illustrates the Ayurvedic approach to hypothyroidism, emphasizing a holistic treatment strategy that addresses the underlying imbalances rather than simply managing the symptoms. It showcases the use of specific herbal formulations and lifestyle modifications tailored to the individual's presentation. The study provides a valuable insight into the potential of Ayurvedic medicine in managing hypothyroidism, but it also highlights the need for more robust research to confirm its efficacy and safety.

Case Study-2: Source: - Monisha P, G Shrinivasa Acharya, Nishanth Pai K, Shrilatha Kamath T. Ayurvedic management of Hypothyroidism - A Case Study. J Ayurveda Integr Med Sci 2022; 1:424-426.

CASE STUDY - 3

This study offers a detailed case study that examines the Ayurvedic management of hypothyroidism in a 50-year-old female patient. The study, published in the *Journal of Ayurveda and Integrative Medical Sciences*, highlights the principles and practices involved in treating hypothyroidism from an Ayurvedic perspective.

CONNECTING HYPOTHYROIDISM TO AYURVEDIC PRINCIPLES

The authors emphasize that while hypothyroidism is not directly mentioned in classical Ayurvedic texts, its symptoms and underlying pathology can be understood within the framework of Ayurvedic principles. They relate the clinical presentation of hypothyroidism to *Kaphaja Nanatmaja Vikaras*, disorders arising from an imbalance in the *Kapha Dosha*.

The case study highlights the similarities between the symptoms of hypothyroidism and those associated with *Kapha* disorders. Symptoms such as *Gurugatrata* (feeling of heaviness), *Alasya* (lethargy), *Tandra* (drowsiness), *Atisthoulya* (obesity or weight gain), and *Atinidra* (excessive sleep) are common to both conditions. This connection suggests that an excess of *Kapha Dosha* might play a role in the development of hypothyroidism.

Further, the case study links hypothyroidism to *Medo Dhatvagni mandya*, a condition characterized by impaired digestive fire responsible for processing *Medo Dhatu* (fat tissue). This impairment is believed to lead to the excessive accumulation of *Medo Dhatu*, contributing to symptoms like weight gain and lethargy.

TREATMENT MODALITIES IN THIS CASE STUDY

The treatment approach adopted in the case study involved a combination of *Shodhana* (purification therapies) and *Shamana* (palliative therapies). This multifaceted approach aims to purify the body, eliminate accumulated toxins, and restore balance to the *Doshas* and *Srotas* (channels).

SHODHANA CHIKITSA

- **Virechana (Therapeutic Purgation)**: *Virechana*, a therapeutic purgation procedure, was administered to eliminate excess *Pitta Dosha*. This procedure involves using specific herbal formulations to induce controlled bowel movements, expelling toxins and rebalancing *Pitta*. The authors explain that *Virechana* is particularly beneficial in cases where *Pitta* is associated with *Kapha*, as it effectively eliminates both *Doshas* from their respective sites.
- **Basti (Therapeutic Enema)**: *Basti*, a therapeutic enema, was administered to further purify and balance the body. Two types of *Basti* were used:
  - **Anuvasana Basti with Sahachar Taila**: An oil-based enema to pacify *Vata Dosha*.
  - **Niruha Basti with Dashamool decoction**: A decoction-based enema to pacify *Pitta* and *Kapha Doshas*. The case study highlights the role of *Basti* in addressing the "thyroid-gut connection." It explains that a significant portion of thyroid function relies on healthy gut bacteria to convert T_4 into T_3, the active thyroid hormone. When digestion is compromised, an overabundance of harmful bacteria can hinder the production of active thyroid hormone. *Basti* is believed to counteract this by its action on the enteric nervous system,

stimulating the central nervous system and the HPT axis, leading to normal thyroid hormone secretion.

SHAMANA CHIKITSA (PALLIATIVE THERAPY)

Following the purification therapies, the patient was prescribed a combination of herbal formulations to manage symptoms and address underlying imbalances. The formulations used were:

- **Tablet Sumedha**: This formulation includes ingredients like *Shankhapushpi*, *Brahmi, Kushmand*, and *Jatamansi* and was prescribed to address neuropsychiatric symptoms such as lack of concentration and fatigue. These ingredients are known for their *Medhya* (nootropic), *Balya* (strengthening), and *Smrutikara* (memory-enhancing) properties.
- **Tablet Amrutarasa**: This formulation, containing ingredients like *Amalaki*, *Shunthi*, *Marich*, and *Pippali*, was given to improve digestion and address symptoms like weight gain and constipation. These ingredients are known for their *Deepana* (appetite-stimulating), *Pachana* (digestive), and *Vata-Kaphahara* (balancing *Vata* and *Kapha Doshas*) actions.
- **Tablet Metaboost**: This formulation, containing ingredients like *Pushkarmoola*, *Guggulu*, *Arjuna*, and *Haritaki*, was prescribed to enhance overall metabolism and regulate digestion and excretion processes.

- **Tablet Granthihar**: This study do not specify the ingredients in this tablet but mention it was administered for two months.

REPORTED OUTCOMES AND FOLLOW-UP

The case study reports that the patient showed significant improvement in her symptoms and thyroid profile after the Ayurvedic treatment. After two months, she experienced relief from tiredness, constipation, and lack of concentration. Her weight reduced by 5 kg, and her thyroid profile showed a notable reduction in TSH levels. The patient continued treatment for a total of six months with no reported recurrence of symptoms.

ANALYZING THE CASE STUDY'S FINDINGS

The authors attribute the positive outcomes to the combined effects of *Shodhana* and *Shamana* therapies. They suggest that *Virechana* effectively addressed constipation, which can impair hormonal clearance and contribute to elevated TSH levels. They also propose that *Basti*, by acting on the enteric nervous system, influences the HPT axis and promotes thyroid hormone secretion.

The case study offers a preliminary exploration of the potential benefits of Ayurvedic medicine in managing hypothyroidism. It showcases how Ayurvedic principles can be applied to understand and address a condition not explicitly described in classical texts. The multimodal approach, combining *Shodhana* and *Shamana* therapies, is presented as an effective way to manage the underlying imbalances and alleviate symptoms. However, further research, particularly large-scale, controlled studies, are needed to validate these findings and establish the efficacy and safety of Ayurvedic treatment for hypothyroidism.

UNDERSTANDING THE CONCEPT OF *SHODHANA* THERAPY

Shodhana therapy, a core component of *Panchakarma*, focuses on eliminating accumulated toxins and imbalances from the body. The sources emphasize the role of *Shodhana* in treating *Bahudoshavastha*, a condition where multiple *Doshas* are aggravated. *Virechana* and *Basti*, as discussed in this study, fall under the umbrella of *Shodhana* therapies.

EXPLORING *VIRECHANA*: THERAPEUTIC PURGATION

Virechana, aimed at eliminating excess *Pitta Dosha*, is discussed in detail within the case study. The procedure involves administering specific herbal formulations that induce controlled bowel movements, purging toxins and restoring balance to *Pitta*. This trial underscore the importance of *Virechana* when *Pitta* is associated with *Kapha*, as seen in the case study, due to its effectiveness in eliminating both *Doshas* from their respective sites.

PREPARATORY PROCEDURES FOR *VIRECHANA*

The case study outlines the preparatory steps involved in *Virechana*, including *Snehana* (internal and external oleation) and *Swedana* (sudation therapy). These preparatory measures aim to prepare the body for the main procedure, facilitating the mobilization and elimination of toxins.

- **Snehana (Internal Oleation):** In the case study, *Snehana* was performed using *Panchatikta Ghrita*, a medicated ghee formulated with herbs known for their penetrating and detoxifying properties. The gradual increase in the dosage of *Panchatikta Ghrita* over several days led to the manifestation of *Snehasiddhi Lakshana*, indicating the body's readiness for *Virechana*.
- **Sarvanga Abhyanga (External Oleation) and Sarvanga Vashpa Swedana (External Sudation)**: Following internal oleation, the patient underwent external oleation with *Bala Taila* and external sudation with a *Dashamool* decoction. These procedures further enhance the mobilization of toxins and prepare the body for purgation.

ADMINISTRATION OF *VIRECHANA* AND ITS EFFECTS

The sources detail the administration of a specific *Virechana* tablet containing herbs like *Haritaki*, *Katuka*, *Trivrit*, and *Snuhikshir*, known for their purgative and *Vata-Kapha Hara* (balancing *Vata* and *Kapha Doshas*) actions. The patient experienced 14 *Vegas* (bowel movements), indicating the effective elimination of toxins.

POST-THERAPY REGIMEN

Following *Virechana*, the patient adhered to *Samsarjan Krama*, a specific post-therapy dietary regimen that gradually reintroduces foods to support recovery and maintain balance.

UNPACKING BASTI: THERAPEUTIC ENEMA

Basti, another crucial *Shodhana* therapy, is highlighted in this study for its role in purifying and balancing the body. Two types of *Basti* were employed in the case study: *Anuvasana Basti* with *Sahachar Taila* and *Niruha Basti* with a *Dashamool* decoction. This study underscore the significance of *Basti* in addressing the "*thyroid-gut connection*," emphasizing its influence on the enteric nervous system and its role in regulating thyroid hormone production.

TYPES OF *BASTI* ADMINISTERED

- *Anuvasana Basti* with *Sahachar Taila*: This oil-based enema is known for its *Vata Dosha*-pacifying properties.
- *Niruha Basti* with *Dashamool* decoction: This decoction-based enema is known for its *Pitta* and *Kapha Dosha*-pacifying properties.

PROPOSED MECHANISMS OF ACTION

The trial suggest that *Basti* exerts its effects through the following mechanisms:

- **Stimulating the Enteric Nervous System**: *Basti* is believed to act on receptors in the enteric nervous system, influencing the central nervous system and subsequently the HPT axis, contributing to normal thyroid hormone secretion.
- **Addressing Gut Dysbiosis**: *Basti* is proposed to counteract gut dysbiosis, an imbalance in gut bacteria that can hinder the conversion of T_4 to T_3, the active thyroid hormone. This action is thought to support optimal thyroid function.

CONCLUDING THOUGHTS ON *PANCHAKARMA* IN THE CASE STUDY

The case study provides a glimpse into the application of two specific *Panchakarma* procedures, *Virechana* and *Basti*, in the management of hypothyroidism. While the study's focus is on the broader Ayurvedic treatment approach, the detailed descriptions of these procedures offer valuable insights into their significance, preparatory measures, and proposed mechanisms of action within the context of the case. However, it is crucial to recognize the limitations of the case study, as discussed in our previous conversation, and the need for further research to validate these findings and establish the efficacy and safety of *Panchakarma* therapies for hypothyroidism.

Case Study-3: Source- Smita Naram, Komal Gawali, Hemang Parekh. Management of Hypothyroidism with Ayurveda - A Case Study. J Ayurveda Integr Med Sci 2024; 3:267-272.

CASE STUDY - 4

This is a detailed case study of a 24-year-old female patient diagnosed with hypothyroidism, focusing on the application and effectiveness of Ayurvedic interventions in her treatment.

PATIENT PRESENTATION AND DIAGNOSIS

The patient initially sought medical attention for a range of symptoms, including irregular menstruation, heaviness throughout the body, fatigue, constipation, and gradual weight gain. These symptoms, alongside diagnostic assessments like ultrasonography and serum TSH level evaluation, led to a diagnosis of hypothyroidism. The ultrasonography also revealed a polycystic ovary syndrome (PCOS)-like presentation, with mildly enlarged bilateral ovaries exhibiting multiple small follicles and increased ovarian stroma.

AYURVEDIC UNDERSTANDING AND TREATMENT APPROACH

This study emphasize that while the term "hypothyroidism" isn't explicitly described in classical Ayurvedic texts, the condition is conceptualized within the framework of *Agni* (digestive fire) and *Dosha* imbalances. The patient's symptoms were attributed to *Agnimandya* (weakened digestive fire) and *Ama* (undigested metabolic waste) accumulation, primarily resulting from dietary and lifestyle factors.

The Ayurvedic treatment approach aimed to:

- Rekindle *Agni*
- Balance *Doshas*, particularly *Kapha* and *Vata*
- Eliminate *Ama*
- Restore proper functioning of *Dhatus* (tissues) and *Srotas* (channels)

THERAPEUTIC INTERVENTIONS

A multi-faceted approach was employed, incorporating the following:

- **Herbal Formulations:** The patient received a combination of herbal formulations, including *Kanchnar Guggulu, Chitrakadi Vati*, tablet *thyrin*, *Kumaryasava*, and a blend of *Haritaki* and *Guduchi churna*, each chosen for its specific properties, such as *Agnideepaka* (digestive fire stimulating), *Strotoshodhak* (channel cleansing), *VataKaphashamaka* (*Vata* and *Kapha* pacifying), and *Granthihar* (tumour reducing).
- **Dietary Modifications:** The patient was advised to adopt dietary changes aligned with Ayurvedic principles, emphasizing easily digestible foods and avoiding those that could aggravate *Kapha*.
- **Panchakarma Therapies:** While not explicitly described in this case study, our previous conversation highlights the role of *Panchakarma* therapies like *Virechana* (therapeutic purgation) and *Basti* (therapeutic enema) in addressing *Dosha* imbalances and purifying the body.

FOLLOW-UP AND OUTCOMES

The patient underwent treatment for five months, with regular follow-ups to monitor progress. Significant improvements were observed in her symptoms, including:

- Relief from constipation within two months
- Improvement in menstrual flow and regularity
- Resolution of heaviness and lethargy by the third follow-up
- Normalized serum TSH levels
- Resolution of multiple small follicles in bilateral ovaries and reduction in ovarian volume as observed through ultrasonography

CONCLUSIONS AND IMPLICATIONS

The case study highlights the potential of **Ayurveda** in managing hypothyroidism. The comprehensive approach, addressing not only the symptoms but also the underlying *Dosha* imbalances and digestive dysfunction, resulted in significant clinical improvements. However, it's important to note that this is a single case report and further research is needed to validate the effectiveness of Ayurvedic interventions for hypothyroidism on a broader scale.

CONCEPTUALIZING HYPOTHYROIDISM IN AYURVEDA

Although "hypothyroidism" as a distinct disease isn't explicitly mentioned in traditional Ayurvedic texts, this study illustrate how

Ayurvedic practitioners understand and approach this condition. They emphasize that hypothyroidism can be viewed through the lens of *Agni* (digestive fire) and *Dosha* imbalances.

- **Agni and Ama:** The case study attributes the patient's hypothyroidism symptoms to *Agnimandya* (weakened digestive fire) and the accumulation of *Ama* (undigested metabolic waste). These imbalances, according to **Ayurveda**, can disrupt the body's natural processes and lead to various health issues.
- **Dosha Imbalances:** This study highlight the role of *Kapha* and *Vata Doshas* in the development of hypothyroidism symptoms. *Kapha*, associated with qualities like heaviness, coldness, and slowness, can contribute to symptoms such as weight gain, lethargy, and constipation. *Vata*, linked to movement and dryness, can manifest as irregular menstruation and anxiety.

AYURVEDIC TREATMENT STRATEGIES IN ACTION

The case study showcases a multi-pronged Ayurvedic treatment approach aimed at restoring balance and addressing the root causes of the patient's hypothyroidism.

- **Herbal Formulations**: The patient was prescribed a combination of Ayurvedic herbal formulations. These formulations were carefully selected based on their traditional properties, targeting specific aspects of the patient's condition. For example, formulations like Kanchnar Guggulu and Chitrakadi Vati were chosen for their Agnideepaka (digestive fire stimulating) and Strotoshodhak (channel cleansing) properties, aiming to rekindle Agni and clear blockages in the body's channels.

- **Dietary Modifications**: Recognizing the impact of diet on ***Dosha*** balance, the patient was advised to make dietary changes. This included avoiding foods thought to aggravate ***Kapha***, such as heavy, oily, and cold foods.
- **Panchakarma Therapies:** While the case study doesn't explicitly detail their use, our previous conversation mentioned the importance of *Panchakarma* therapies, specifically *Virechana* (therapeutic purgation) and *Basti* (therapeutic enema). These therapies are believed to eliminate toxins, pacify *Doshas*, and restore balance within the body.

OBSERVING TREATMENT OUTCOMES

The case study documents positive outcomes following the five-month Ayurvedic intervention, including:

- **Relief from symptoms**: The patient experienced a reduction in constipation, improved menstrual flow and regularity, and resolution of heaviness and lethargy.
- **Normalization of serum TSH levels**: The patient's TSH levels, a key indicator of thyroid function, returned to the normal range.

- **Improvement in ovarian health**: Ultrasonography revealed a resolution of multiple small follicles in the ovaries and a decrease in ovarian volume, suggesting an improvement in PCOS-related concerns.

Case Study-4: Source- Kapoor AB, Raturi S. Role of Ayurveda in the management of hypothyroidism A case report. Indian J Ayurveda Integr Med 2022; 8:99 103.

CASE STUDY - 5

This study offer a focused look at Ayurvedic treatment methods, specifically through a randomized comparative pilot clinical trial examining the efficacy of *Vyoshadi Guggulu* and *Shadushana Churna* in managing subclinical hypothyroidism (SCH).

AYURVEDIC TREATMENT STRATEGIES

The Ayurvedic treatment approach aims to address the root cause of SCH, which is *Agnimandya*. Two specific formulations, *Vyoshadi Guggulu* and *Shadushana Churna*, are highlighted for their potential in managing SCH.

- **Targeting Agni and Microchannels:** Both *Vyoshadi Guggulu* and *Shadushana Churna* possess properties that stimulate digestion and metabolism (*Deepana* and *Pachana*), clear microchannels (*Srotoshodhaka*), reduce fat (*Medohara*), and scrape away fat and lipid contents (*Lekhana*). By improving Agni and addressing the vitiation of microchannels that carry lipids and nutrients, these formulations are believed to correct the underlying pathology of SCH.

CLINICAL TRIAL INSIGHTS

The pilot clinical trial involved 30 patients with SCH randomly divided into two groups. Group A received *Vyoshadi Guggulu* (6 g twice daily), while Group B received *Shadushana Churna* (3 g twice daily) for 60 days. The primary outcome measure was the change in serum TSH levels, while secondary outcomes included changes in body mass index (BMI) and safety assessments.

KEY FINDINGS:

- **Reduction in Serum TSH:** Both Vyoshadi Guggulu and Shadushana Churna led to statistically significant reductions in serum TSH levels (16.61% and 26.29%, respectively).
- **Decrease in BMI:** Both formulations also significantly reduced BMI.
- **Safety Profile:** No adverse drug reactions were reported, and liver and kidney function tests remained within normal limits, indicating the safety of both formulations at the tested doses.

MODES OF ACTION:

The therapeutic effects of *Vyoshadi Guggulu* and *Shadushana Churna* can be attributed to their specific ingredients and their pharmacological properties.

- **Vyoshadi Guggulu:** The ingredients in *Vyoshadi Guggulu*, such as ginger (*Shunthi*), long pepper (*Pippali*), and guggulu (*Commiphora Mukul*) possess properties that stimulate digestive fire, reduce *Kapha* and fat, and potentially stimulate thyroid hormone release.
- **Shadushana Churna:** The ingredients in *Shadushana Churna*, including black pepper (*Pippali*), ginger, and long pepper, are known for their digestive stimulating, *Kapha* reducing, and metabolism-boosting effects.

THE MECHANISMS OF ACTION OF VYOSHADI GUGGULU AND SHADUSHANA CHURNA

Both *Vyoshadi Guggulu* and *Shadushana Churna* are composed of herbs that possess specific properties aimed at correcting the imbalances associated with SCH.

- **Stimulating Digestion and Metabolism:** These formulations contain ingredients known for their digestive stimulating (*Deepana*) and metabolic enhancing (*Pachana*) properties. This helps improve the body's ability to process food and generate energy, counteracting *Agnimandya*.
- **Clearing Microchannels:** They also exhibit *Srotoshodhaka* properties, which means they help clear blockages in the body's microchannels. This allows for the proper flow of nutrients and

energy, restoring balance to the Dhatu-Sara.

- **Reducing Fat and Lipids:** Both formulations include herbs with *Medohara* and *Lekhana* properties, which help reduce excess fat and lipids. This is particularly relevant as weight gain is a common symptom of SCH.

By addressing *Agnimandya* and the vitiation of microchannels, these formulations aim to rectify the underlying pathology of SCH.

KEY FINDINGS FROM THE CLINICAL TRIAL:

- **Significant Reduction in Serum TSH Levels:** Both *Vyoshadi Guggulu* and *Shadushana Churna* led to statistically significant reductions in serum TSH levels. Group A experienced a 16.61% decrease, while Group B showed a 26.29% decrease.
- **BMI Reduction:** Both formulations also resulted in a significant decrease in BMI. Vyoshadi Guggulu led to a 1.80% reduction, and Shadushana Churna led to a 1.36% reduction.
- **Favourable Safety Profile:** No adverse drug reactions were reported during the study, and liver and kidney function tests remained normal, indicating the safety of both formulations at the tested doses.

INTERPRETING THE RESULTS

The findings of this pilot study suggest that both *Vyoshadi Guggulu* and *Shadushana Churna* may have potential as treatment options for

SCH. The observed reductions in serum TSH levels and BMI, coupled with the absence of adverse effects, are encouraging.

However, it is important to acknowledge the limitations of the study, particularly the small sample size. Larger, more rigorous clinical trials with longer follow-up periods are essential to confirm these initial findings and establish the long-term efficacy and safety of these Ayurvedic formulations in the management of SCH.

Future research could also explore the differential effects of *Vyoshadi Guggulu* and *Shadushana Churna* in specific subpopulations of SCH patients, such as those who are obese versus non-obese. This would help tailor treatment recommendations based on individual characteristics and needs.

CONCLUSION

This is a compelling case for considering Ayurvedic approaches to SCH management. The understanding of SCH as a manifestation of *Agnimandya* and the use of targeted herbal formulations like *Vyoshadi Guggulu* and *Shadushana Churna* highlight the holistic and individualized nature of Ayurvedic medicine. While further research is needed to solidify the evidence base, the initial findings offer promising avenues for exploring safe and effective treatments for SCH.

Case Study-5: Source:-Sharma VB, Padhar BC, Meena HM, Mathur SK.Efficacy of Vyoshadi Guggulu and Shadushana Churna in the management of subclinical hypothyroidism: An open labelled randomized comparative pilot clinical trial. AYU 2022; 41:181-7

CONCLUSIONS FROM THE CASE STUDIES

The several conclusions about the application of **Ayurveda** in managing hypothyroidism. Here are some key takeaways:

- Ayurvedic treatments, particularly those focused on *Shodhana* and *Shamana Chikitsa*, can lead to significant improvements in both subjective symptoms and objective measures like thyroid hormone levels. The case studies presented in this study consistently demonstrate positive outcomes for patients undergoing Ayurvedic treatment for hypothyroidism. For instance, the study described in this trial noted a 60% improvement in the patient's condition, including significant reductions in weight, fatigue, hair loss, dry skin, and indigestion, accompanied by positive changes in their thyroid profile. Similarly, this study reports a case of complete symptom resolution after six months of Ayurvedic treatment, including weight loss and a notable decrease in TSH levels. These positive findings suggest that Ayurvedic interventions can effectively address the multifaceted nature of hypothyroidism, targeting both the underlying imbalances and the resulting symptoms.

- *Kshara Basti* emerges as a potentially effective and patient-friendly treatment modality, especially in cases associated with *Ama*. This study highlights the successful application of *Kshara Basti* in a patient with subclinical hypothyroidism and rheumatoid arthritis. The study emphasizes the importance of addressing *Ama* in autoimmune conditions like hypothyroidism. The authors note that *Kshara Basti*, being relatively easy to administer and not requiring *Snehapana* (internal oleation) or *Samsarjana* (specific dietary regimen), could be a preferable treatment option for patients who find these procedures unpleasant. This suggests that *Kshara Basti* could be a valuable addition to the therapeutic arsenal for managing hypothyroidism, particularly in individuals with a predominance of *Ama*.
- Specific herbal formulations like *Vyoshadi Guggulu* and *Shadushana Churna* show promise in reducing serum TSH levels and BMI in subclinical hypothyroidism. The pilot clinical trial described in this study demonstrates the statistically significant efficacy of both *Vyoshadi Guggulu* and *Shadushana Churna* in lowering TSH levels and BMI in patients with subclinical hypothyroidism. The study also highlights the safety of these formulations, with no reported adverse effects during the trial period. These findings suggest that these specific herbal remedies could play a role in managing early stages of

hypothyroidism, potentially preventing its progression to overt hypothyroidism and addressing associated metabolic concerns like weight gain.

Further research is necessary to validate these findings, establish optimal treatment protocols, and explore the underlying mechanisms of action of Ayurvedic remedies in hypothyroidism. While the various studies provide encouraging evidence for the potential of Ayurveda in managing hypothyroidism, they also acknowledge the need for more robust scientific investigation. The review article in this section stresses the importance of conducting larger clinical trials to confirm existing findings and optimize treatment durations. It also calls for more targeted research to identify the specific mechanisms through which Ayurvedic herbs exert their beneficial effects, whether at the level of the thyroid gland itself or through peripheral tissues involved in thyroid hormone production and metabolism. Such rigorous research is crucial for establishing the scientific validity of Ayurvedic interventions and integrating them effectively into modern healthcare practices.

- $$$ -

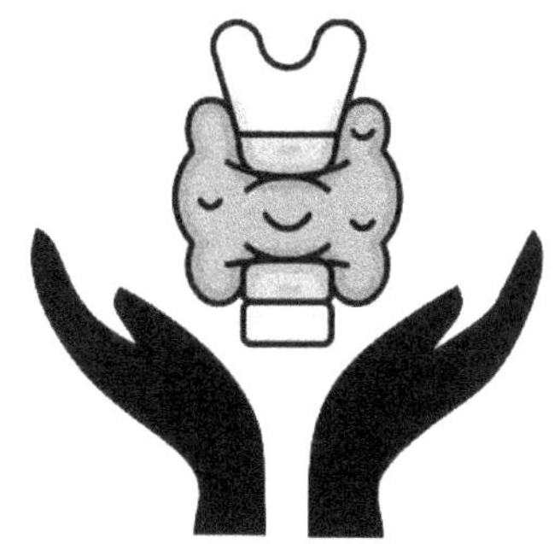

Author Profile

DR. AJAY KUMAR

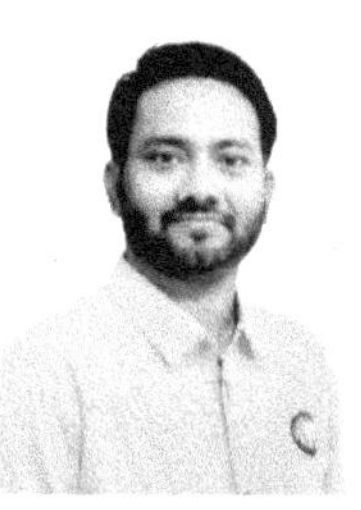

Dr. Ajay Kumar is currently working as an Assistant Professor in the Department of Kayachikitsa and Panchakarma at Government Post Graduate Ayurveda College and Hospital, Varanasi. He has completed B.A.M.S. in 2005 from the same college and completed M.D. and Ph. D. in Kayachikitsa from Banaras Hindu University. His main areas of specialization are hypertension, cardio-respiratory and diabetes. Here's more about his work and contributions:

EDUCATIONAL AND PROFESSIONAL BACKGROUND

- **Position**: Assistant Professor, Department of Kayachikitsa and Panchakarma.
- **Institution**: Government Post Graduate Ayurveda College and

Hospital, Varanasi.

- **Experience**: Over 15 years in Ayurveda practice and education.

AREAS OF SPECIALIZATION

Dr. Gupta treats a wide range of ailments using traditional Ayurvedic methods, including:

- Chronic diseases such as diabetes, hypertension, arthritis, and kidney issues.
- Skin disorders like psoriasis and eczema.
- Gastrointestinal problems such as acidity and IBS.
- Male infertility.
- Stress and lifestyle-related disorders.

PUBLISHED WORKS

Dr. Gupta has authored several books to promote Ayurveda and holistic health:

- "बीमारियों को हराएंगे" - Focuses on overcoming diseases through Ayurveda.
- "मधुमेह" - A guide to managing diabetes naturally.
- "वनौषधि दर्पण" - Encyclopedia of medicinal plants and herbs.
- "चरक सार संग्रह" (Co-authored with Dr. Tina Singhal) - A concise collection of Charaka Samhita principles.

- "Male Infertility & Management" (Co-authored with Dr. Tina Singhal) - Ayurvedic solutions to male infertility.
- "Hypertension & Ayurveda" - Integrating Ayurvedic remedies for hypertension.
- "सुश्रुत तत्व प्रदीपिका" (Co-authored with Dr. Tina Singhal) - Insights from Sushruta Samhita.
- "Diabetes- Who Knows More Lives More" - Integrating Ayurvedic remedies for Diabetes.

About 40 research papers have been published in International and National level journals & more than 300 health related articles have been written for national level Newspapers. He has presented guest lectures in more than 30 International and National level seminars, and has also organized several seminars.

DIGITAL PRESENCE

- YouTube Channels-
  - **Arogya Street**: For health education and awareness.
  - **AYUSHVANI**: Sharing Ayurvedic knowledge and remedies.

WEBSITE

For further details, you can visit his official website:

- www.drajayg.in
- www.drajayg.wordpress.com

DR. TINA SINGHAL

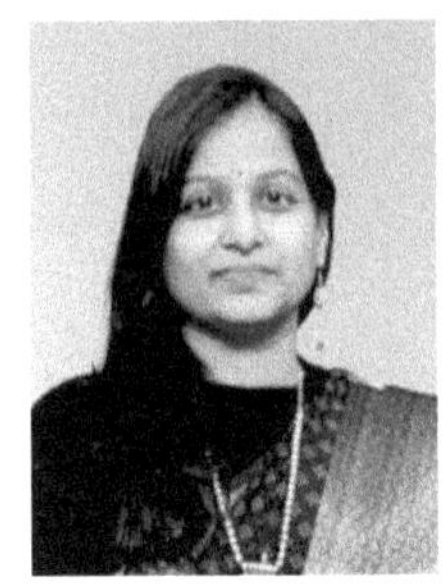

Dr. Tina Singhal is a Lecturer in the Department of Rachana Sharir (Anatomy) at the Government Ayurvedic College and Hospital in Varanasi, India. She completed her Bachelor of Ayurvedic Medicine and Surgery (BAMS) from the same institution and pursued her M.D. in Rachana Sharir at Banaras Hindu University (BHU), Varanasi. Additionally, she holds a Ph.D. in Rachana Sharir from Sampurnanand Sanskrit University, Varanasi. Dr. Singhal has been serving as a Lecturer since 2012, and has 12 years of teaching experience.

She has contributed to the field of Ayurveda through publications, including works on Hypertension, Diabetes, Kidney Disease etc. Dr. Singhal is also active on ResearchGate, where she shares her research and connects with fellow scholars.

For students and practitioners, Dr. Singhal offers educational content on Ayurveda. Her Many lectures on Anatomy & Charak Samhita is available on YouTube Channel “AYUSHVANI”.

EDUCATIONAL AND PROFESSIONAL BACKGROUND

- **Position**: Assistant Professor, Department of Rachana Sharir.
- **Institution**: Government Post Graduate Ayurveda College and Hospital, Varanasi.

- **Experience**: Over 12 years in Ayurveda practice and education.

PUBLISHED WORKS

Dr. Tina Singhal has authored several books to promote Ayurveda and holistic health:

- बीमारियों को हराएंगे
- वनौषधि दर्पण
- चरक सार संग्रह
- Male Infertility & Management
- सुश्रुत तत्व प्रदीपिका

About 35 research papers have been published in International and National level journals. She has presented guest lectures in more than 30 International and National level seminars, and has also organized several seminars.

DR. PRATIMA YADAV

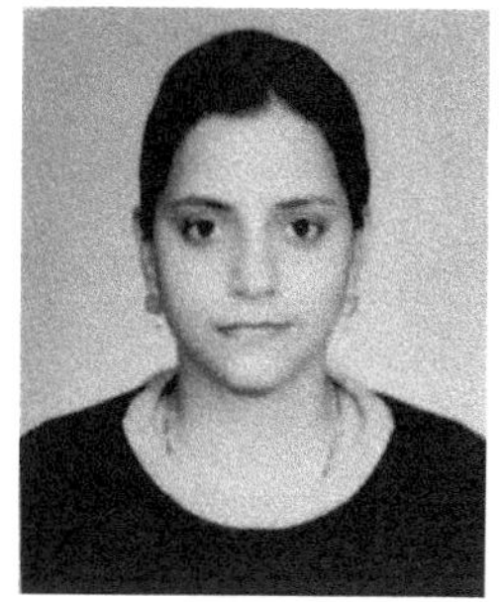

Dr Pratima Yadav (MD Panchakarma) originally hails from Mainpuri, Uttar Pradesh. She passed the Ayurvedacharya(B.A.M.S) degree course in 2017 from State Ayurvedic College and Hospital, Lucknow which was conducted by the University of Lucknow. She has worked as an intern in Balrampur district hospital, lucknow. She completed MD(Panchakarma) in 2023 from Govt. PG Ayurvedic College and Hospital, Varanasi.

The author loves to read and write as well. Apart from this book, she has written and published approx 10 articles in different international research journals. Currently she is working as a medical officer (Community health).

DR. ABHISHEK YADAV

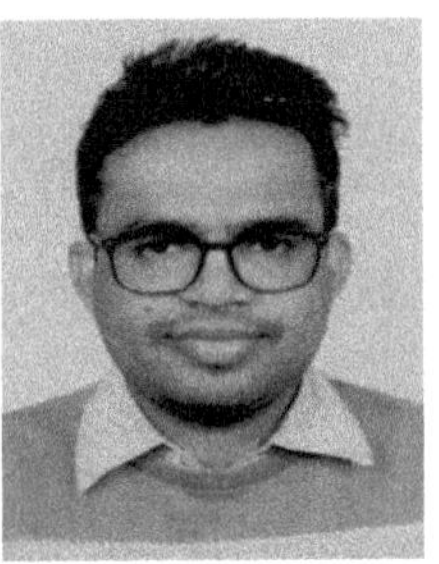

Dr. Abhishek Yadav, a qualified BAMS graduate from Swami Kalyan Dev Ranjiya Ayurveda College, Muzaffarnagar, U.P., completed his studies in the batch of 2009. He pursued his postgraduate studies at the Govt. P.G. Ayurvedic College and Hospital, Varanasi, U.P., earning an MD degree in 2018.

Dr. Yadav has a particular interest in the management of neurological disorders, including Parkinson's Disease and Cerebellar Ataxia, and has contributed to the field through his research paper titled *A Review on Parkinson's Disease and Cerebellar Ataxia and its Management through Sarvangdhara*.

Qualification: BAMS, MD (Ayurveda)

Specialization: Parkinson's Disease, Cerebellar Ataxia, Panchakarma

ACADEMIC BACKGROUND

- **BAMS**: Swami Kalyan Dev Ranjiya Ayurveda College, Muzaffarnagar, U.P. (Batch: 2009)
- **MD/MS**: Govt. P.G. Ayurvedic College and Hospital, Varanasi, U.P. (Batch: 2018)

Current Role

- **Present Working** as Medical Officer in UP Govt.

Publications

- **Research Paper**:
  A Review on Parkinson's Disease and Cerebellar Ataxia and its Management through Sarvangdhara

DR. JYOTI KAUSHIK

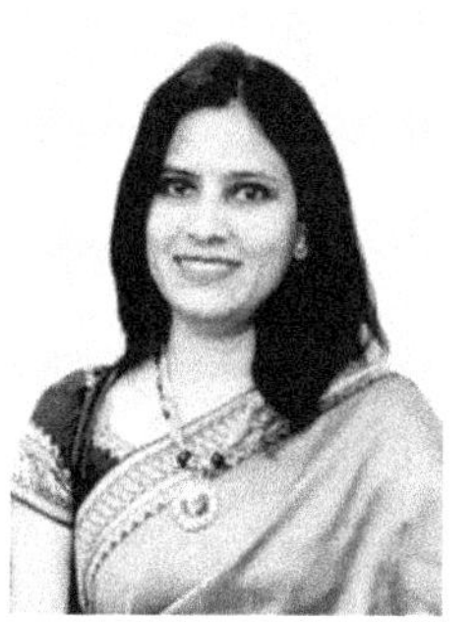

Dr. Jyoti Kaushik completed her Bachelor of Ayurvedic Medicine and Surgery (BAMS) at MSM Institute of Ayurveda, Khanpur Kalan, Sonipat, as part of the 2013 batch. She pursued her postgraduate studies at Government Ayurveda College and Hospital, Varanasi, earning her MD/MS degree in the batch of 2020-2021. Currently, she is working as a General Practitioner at Santosh Medical and Dental Hospital in Gurgaon.

Dr. Kaushik has made significant contributions to Ayurvedic literature and research. She published an article titled *Agni and its Clinical Importance in Ayurveda* in the book *Compendium of Bio-fire in Ayurveda (Agni Vyapar)* by AIASPGA, New Delhi, 2022. Additionally, she has authored numerous research papers, including studies on Virechana Karma in Diabetes Mellitus, the preventive and therapeutic effects of Yogasana and Pranayama in hypertension, and the roles of Agnikarma and Marma therapy in frozen shoulder management. Her works also explore Ayurvedic perspectives on diabetes management, the use of Vaitarana Basti in rheumatoid arthritis, and the enhancement of mobility and muscle strength in the elderly.

Beyond her academic achievements, Dr. Kaushik has participated in several national and international seminars and webinars. These include events on Ayurvedic Garbhasanskar, spinal diseases, scientific writing, and evidence-based Ayurveda. Notably, she volunteered in a Continuing Medical Education program for doctors on Panchakarma, organized by the PG Department of Panchakarma at Government Ayurveda College and Hospital, Varanasi.

ACADEMIC BACKGROUND

- **BAMS**: MSM Institute of Ayurveda, Khanpur Kalan, Sonipat (Batch: 2013).

- **MD/MS**: Government Ayurveda College and Hospital, Varanasi (Batch: 2020-2021).

CURRENT ROLE

- General Practitioner at Santosh Medical and Dental Hospital, Gurgaon.

PUBLICATIONS

- Book Contribution:

  Agni and its Clinical Importance in Ayurveda in *Compendium of Bio-fire in Ayurveda (Agni Vyapar)* by AIASPGA, New Delhi, 2022 (ISBN: 978-93-94582-55-2).

- Research Papers:
  - *Clinical Effect of Virechana Karma in Madhumeha w.s.r to Diabetes Mellitus - A Case Study* (Journal of Ayurveda and Integrated Medical Sciences, Vol. 8, Issue 6, June 2023).
  - *Preventive and Therapeutic Effect of Yogasana and Pranayama in the Patient of Hypertension: An Overview* (IAMJ Journal, Vol. 11, Issue 09, September 2023).
  - *Role of Agnikarma and Marma Therapy in Avabahuka w.s.r. to Frozen Shoulder - A Case Study* (IAMJ Journal, Vol. 11, Issue 11, January 2023).

- *Diabetes in Elderly and its Management from Ayurvedic and Modern Approach – A Review* (IRJAY Journal, Vol. 6, Issue 9, September 2023).
- *Conceptual Overview of Efficacy of Virechana Karma in Madhumeha w.s.r. to Diabetes Mellitus Type – 2* (IJRAP Journal, Vol. 14, Issue 1, 2023).
- *Role of Vaitarana Basti in Management of Amavata w.s.r. to Rheumatoid Arthritis – A Case Study* (IRJAY Journal, Vol. 4, Issue 12, December 2021).
- *Role of Ayurveda in Enhancement of Mobility and Muscle Strength of the Elderly – A Review* (IRJAY Journal, Vol. 7, Issue 6, June 2024).

SEMINARS AND WEBINARS ATTENDED

1. National Webinar on *Ayurvedic Garbhasanskar*, 8 February 2022, MSM Institute of Ayurveda, Sonipat, Haryana.
2. International Conference on *Bharatiya Sangyaharak Association*, 20-21 March 2022, U.P. State Branch, A.A.I.M., and Government Ayurvedic P.G. College & Hospital, Varanasi.

3. National Webinar on *Role of Ayurveda in Spinal Diseases w.s.r. (Kati Grah-Slip Disc)*, 7 April 2022, The Kairali Ayurvedic Group.

4. International Webinar on *Synopsis & Scientific Writing*, 17-24 May 2021, SDM College of Ayurveda & Hospital, Karnataka.

5. Sensitization Program on *Ayurvedic Aahar* by Rashtriya Ayurveda Vidyapeeth, New Delhi, 4 March 2023.

6. International Conference and Workshop on *Evidence-based Ayurveda and Live Practical Demonstration of Ayurveda Upkrama*, 11-12 January 2023, Vrindavan, U.P.

7. Volunteered in Continuing Medical Education for Doctors on Panchakarma, 22-27 November 2021, PG Department of Panchakarma, Government Ayurveda College and Hospital, Varanasi.

DR. SURABHI SINGH

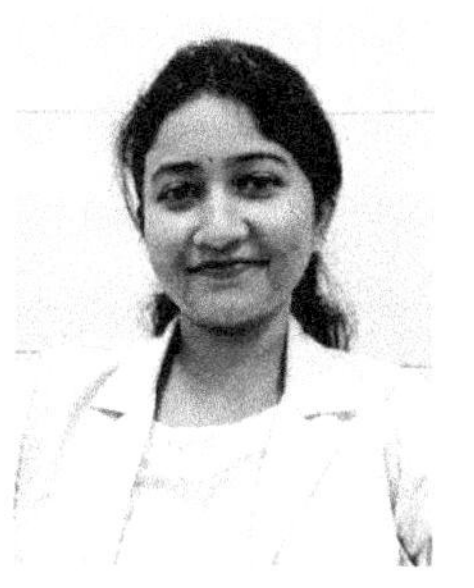

Dr. Surabhi Singh completed her Bachelor of Ayurvedic Medicine and Surgery (BAMS) from U.A.U Gurukul Campus, Haridwar, Uttarakhand, in the batch of 2016. She pursued her postgraduate studies at Govt. P.G. Ayurvedic College and Hospital, Varanasi, U.P., earning her MD degree in Panchakarma in 2022. Dr. Singh has contributed to Ayurvedic research through her paper titled *A Review on Management of Vataja Shirorog w.s.r. to Tension-Type Headache through Dashmooladi Siddha Ksheerdhara and Oral Administration*.

ACADEMIC BACKGROUND

- BAMS: U.A.U Gurukul Campus, Haridwar, Uttarakhand (Batch: 2016).
- MD/MS: Govt. P.G. Ayurvedic College and Hospital, Varanasi, U.P. (Batch: 2022).

CURRENT ROLE

Pursuing M.D. in Panchakarma.

RESEARCH PAPERS

A Review on Management of Vataja Shirorog w.s.r. to Tension-Type Headache through Dashmooladi Siddha Ksheerdhara and Oral Administration.

-$$$-

www.ingramcontent.com/pod-product-compliance
Ingram Content Group UK Ltd.
Pitfield, Milton Keynes, MK11 3LW, UK
UKHW061132310726
14090UKWH00035B/781